microwaving light meals & snacks

microwave cooking library®

by barbara methven

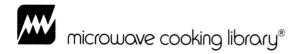
microwave cooking library®

The recipes in this cookbook reflect contemporary eating styles. Whether you want a tasty munch between meals, fun-to-drink refreshments for entertaining, or a light but interesting lunch or supper, prepare them easily in your microwave oven.

Use these versatile recipes with imagination. Some of the snacks, like the Mediterranean Snack Platter, the Cheese Crisps or the individual Snack Pizzas make excellent light meals. Among the beverages, a few quench your thirst, while others are filling enough for a snack. The sweet snacks provide taste appeal without being too rich or sugary; use them as desserts, too. Meatless dishes serve as a vegetarian main dish or supplement protein as a side dish.

If you think snacks and light meals are short on nutrition and heavy on calories, check the nutrition chart on pages 152 and 153. Used wisely, these recipes help you fit snacks and light meals into a sensible health-and-weight-maintenance life-style.

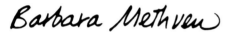

Barbara Methven

CREDITS:
Design & Production: Cy DeCosse Incorporated
Senior Art Director: Bill Nelson
Art Director: Oksana Haliw
Managing Editor: Reneé Dignan
Project Manager: Melissa Erickson
Home Economists: Jill Crum, Peggy Ramette, Kathy Weber
Consultants: Lynn Bachman, Patricia Godfrey, R.D.
Recipe Editor: Susan Meyers
Production Manager: Jim Bindas
Assistant Production Manager: Julie Churchill
Typesetting: Linda Schloegel, Jennie Smith
Production Staff: Janice Cauley, Joe Fahey, Carol Ann Kevan, Yelena Konrardy, Christi Maybee, David Schelitzche, Greg Wallace, Nik Wogstad
Studio Manager: Cathleen Shannon
Photographers: Rex Irman, Tony Kubat, John Lauenstein, Mark Macemon, Mette Nielsen
Food Stylists: Melinda Hutchison, Amy Peterson, Sue Sinon, Ann Stuart
Color Separations: Spectrum, Inc.
Printing: R. R. Donnelley & Sons (0188)

Additional volumes in the Microwave Cooking Library series are available from the publisher:

- Basic Microwaving
- Recipe Conversion for Microwave
- Microwaving Meats
- Microwave Baking & Desserts
- Microwaving Meals in 30 Minutes
- Microwaving on a Diet
- Microwaving Fruits & Vegetables
- Microwaving Convenience Foods
- Microwaving for Holidays & Parties
- Microwaving for One & Two
- The Microwave & Freezer
- 101 Microwaving Secrets
- Microwaving Light & Healthy
- Microwaving Poultry & Seafood
- Microwaving America's Favorites
- Microwaving Fast & Easy Main Dishes
- More Microwaving Secrets

CY DE COSSE INCORPORATED
Chairman: Cy DeCosse
President: James B. Maus
Executive Vice President: William B. Jones

Library of Congress Cataloging-in-Publication Data.

Methven, Barbara.
   Microwaving light meals & snacks.

(Microwave cooking library)

Includes index.
1. Microwave cookery. 2. Cookery (Appetizers). I. Title. II. Title: Microwaving light meals & snacks. III. Series.
TX832.M3977   1988   641.8'12   87-30482
ISBN 0-86573-555-7
ISBN 0-86573-556-5 (pbk.)

Published by Prentice Hall Press
A Division of Simon & Schuster, Inc., New York
ISBN 0-13-582172-X

Contents

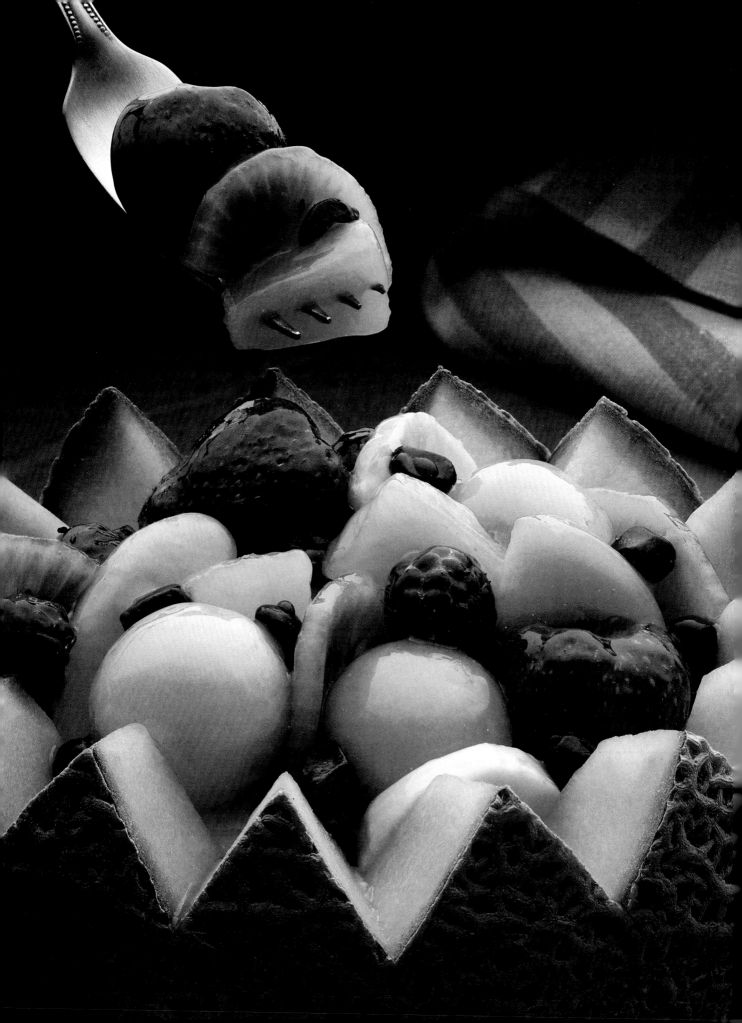

What You Need To Know Before You Start

Today health- and weight-conscious people eat lighter meals, and they recognize that snacking need not be harmful. Our grandparents consumed at least three heavy, hearty meals a day, but their life-styles were such that they utilized more calories through heavy physical labor. Today's active life-styles and hectic schedules encourage people to choose their snacks as wisely as they select their meals to achieve a full day's sound, well-balanced nutrition.

A preference for smaller meals is not limited to dieters. Those of us who follow a three-meals-a-day schedule are eating basic breakfasts, light lunches and simple suppers. Some nutritionists endorse the practice of consuming several well-balanced mini-meals, spaced throughout the day, as a way of keeping the body steadily, but not overly, fueled. Snack lovers maintain satisfactory nutrition by avoiding empty calories and balancing an occasional high-calorie snack with lean meals.

HOW TO USE THIS BOOK

This is not a diet book. The recipes are for delicious, sensible, but not exclusively low-calorie, meals and snacks. Portions are adequate, not excessive. Emphasis is on eye appeal and fresh taste. The recipes avoid cloying sweets or rich sauces. The Snacks and Munchies section provides appetizers and snacks for entertaining or casual nibbling. Many of them can also serve as simple lunches for one to four persons. Beverages include light refreshments as well as substantial liquids to satisfy mid-day or late-night hunger. For those who prefer sweets between meals, the Fruits and Sweet Snacks chapter offers appealing, just-sweet-enough fork and finger foods. You'll enjoy some of them as desserts, too. Salads, Soups and Sandwiches remain popular choices for lunches. The new ideas in this section will provide variety, even if you lunch on these foods daily. The last four sections offer lean entrées for light meals. The recipes reflect contemporary preferences for poultry, fish, seafood, lean meats and high-energy complex carbohydrates.

NUTRITION CHART

For your convenience, the chart on pages 152 and 153 provides information on nutritional values. The chart is arranged according to page number and lists the calorie, protein, carbohydrate, fat and sodium values for a single serving of each recipe. While exchanges are not listed, persons following an exchange diet can, with the assistance of a Registered Dietitian, calculate the exchanges from this information.

The analysis does not include variations, optional ingredients or garnishes. If an unspecified amount of hot cooked rice is listed as an ingredient needed to complete a dish, the nutritional values include a half-cup serving. Where approximate weights or measures are given, such as 2½ to 3 pounds of chicken, the analysis is based on the greater amount.

If a recipe calls for a marinade, the way the marinade is used determines the amount included in the analysis. If the marinade is used as a baste during cooking, the analysis covers the entire amount. The nutritional values include 25% of a marinade that is drained and discarded before microwaving.

Where the recipe provides a flexible number of servings, such as 4 to 6 or 6 to 8, the nutritional analysis is based on the larger number of servings.

For recipes that list total quantities rather than single portions, the following is a base for serving size:

Dips — 2 tablespoons per serving
Appetizers — 2 per serving
Kabobs — 1 per serving
Snack mixes — 1 cup per serving

Using this information as a guide, you can choose snacks and light meals that combine to provide sound nutrition, while you avoid foods that do not fit your personal dietary requirements.

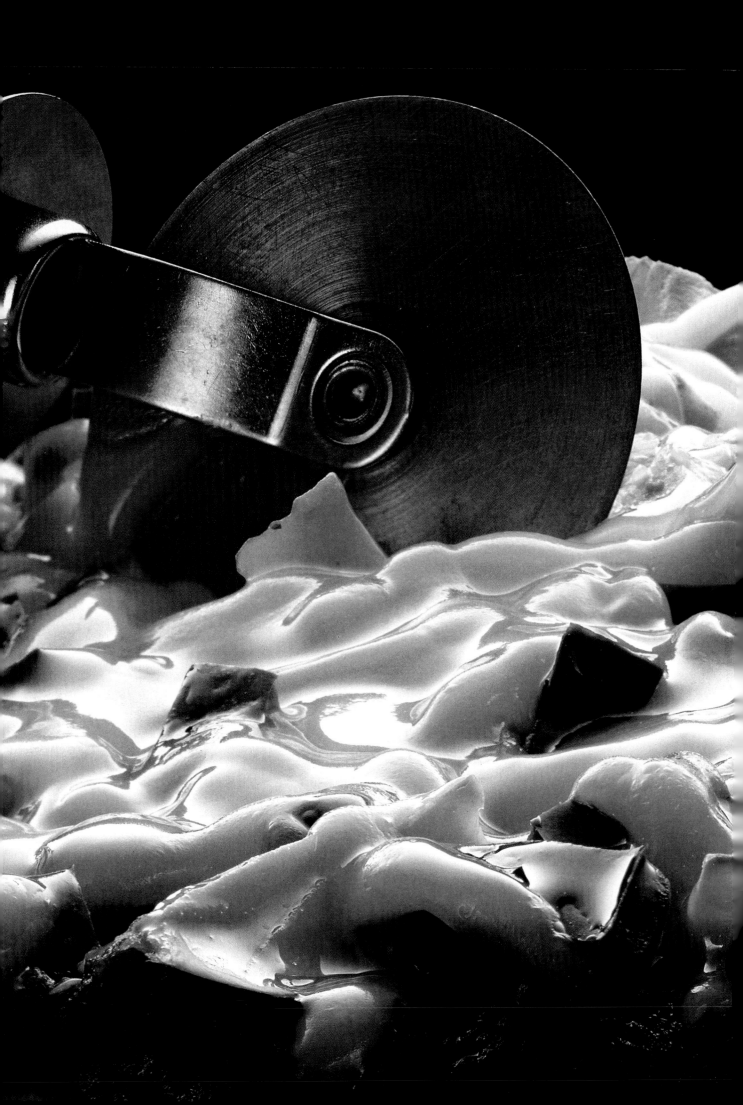

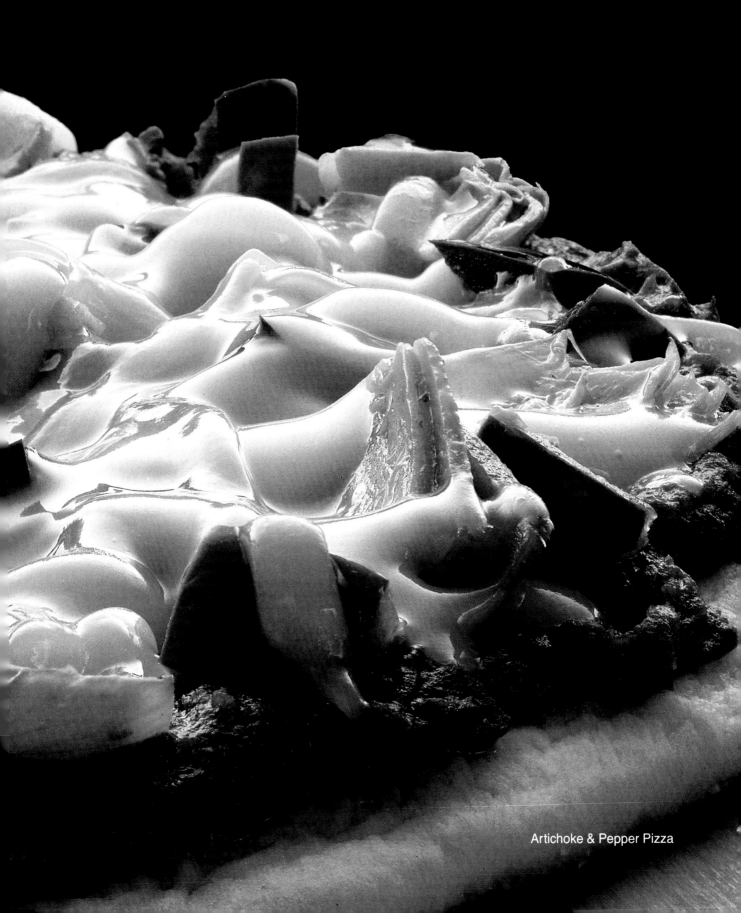

Snacks & Munchies

Artichoke & Pepper Pizza

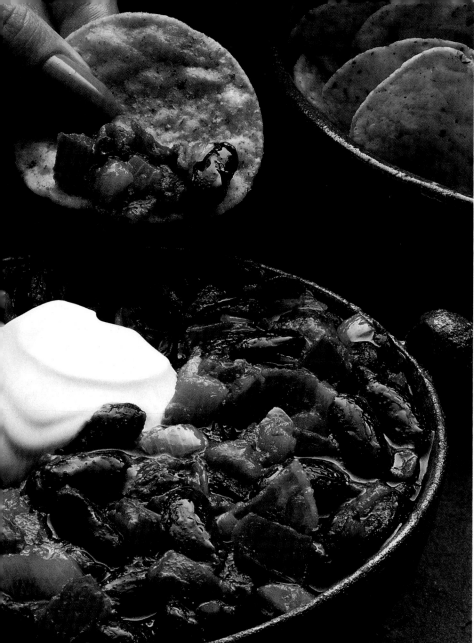

Bean & Salsa Dip

3 slices bacon, cut up
1 small onion, chopped
1 can (16 oz.) dark red kidney
  beans, rinsed and drained,
  divided
⅔ cup salsa
1 small tomato, seeded and
  chopped

About 2½ cups

Place bacon in 1-quart casserole. Cover. Microwave at High for 4 to 6 minutes, or until bacon is brown, stirring once. With slotted spoon, remove bacon to paper towels. Crumble and set aside.

Add onion to bacon fat. Re-cover. Microwave at High for 1½ to 2½ minutes, or until onion is tender. Mash ⅓ cup beans. Add mashed beans and salsa to onion. Mix well. Add bacon, remaining beans and tomato. Mix well. Re-cover. Microwave at High for 3 to 5 minutes, or until dip is hot. Top with sour cream, if desired. Serve warm with tortilla chips.

Broccoli Cheese Dip

2 cups coarsely chopped fresh
  broccoli
½ cup sliced fresh mushrooms
2 tablespoons finely chopped
  onion
2 tablespoons water
1 cup small curd cottage
  cheese
¼ cup mayonnaise
¼ cup grated Parmesan cheese
¼ teaspoon salt
¼ teaspoon lemon pepper
  seasoning
Grated Parmesan cheese
Paprika

About 2 cups

In 1-quart casserole, combine broccoli, mushrooms, onion and water. Cover. Microwave at High for 3 to 4 minutes, or until broccoli is tender-crisp, stirring once. Drain. Set aside.

Place cottage cheese, mayonnaise, ¼ cup Parmesan cheese, salt and lemon pepper in food processor or blender. Process until smooth. Stir cottage cheese mixture into broccoli mixture. Sprinkle with Parmesan cheese and paprika. Microwave, uncovered, at 70% (Medium High) for 1½ to 2½ minutes, or just until dip is hot. Serve warm with crackers or corn chips.

Cucumber Dip ▶

1 large cucumber (about 12 oz.), peeled and seeded
2 teaspoons water
1 teaspoon dried mint flakes
1 teaspoon lime juice
1 pkg. (3 oz.) cream cheese
1 container (8 oz.) plain low-fat yogurt
¼ cup shredded carrot
1 tablespoon snipped fresh parsley
¾ teaspoon seasoned salt
⅛ teaspoon cayenne

About 2 cups

Shred cucumber onto several layers of paper towel. Set aside to drain. In small mixing bowl, combine water, mint flakes and lime juice. Microwave at High for 30 to 45 seconds, or until hot.

Add cream cheese. Microwave at High for 15 to 30 seconds, or until cream cheese softens. Add cucumber and remaining ingredients. Mix well. Cover and chill for at least 2 hours to blend flavors. Serve with vegetables for dipping.

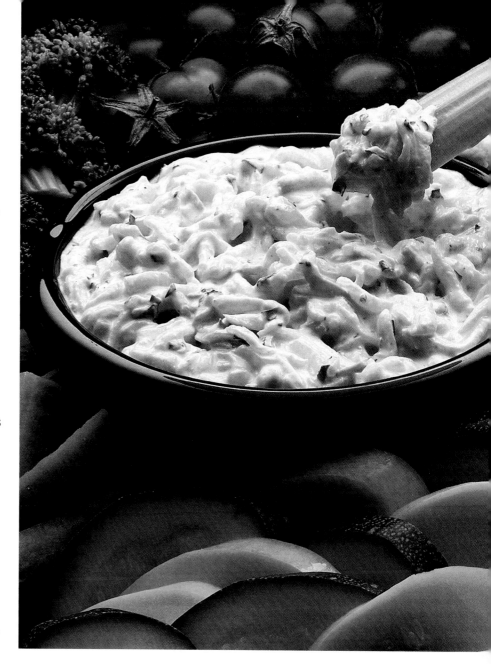

Hummus

¼ cup fresh lemon juice, divided
¼ cup plus 2 tablespoons water, divided
2 tablespoons sesame seed
1 teaspoon vegetable oil
¼ teaspoon sesame oil
½ cup chopped onion
1 clove garlic, minced
1 can (15 oz.) garbanzo beans, rinsed and drained
Snipped fresh parsley (optional)

About 1⅔ cups

In blender, combine 1 teaspoon lemon juice, 2 tablespoons water, the sesame seed, vegetable oil and sesame oil. Process until smooth. Place mixture in 1-quart casserole. Add remaining lemon juice, remaining ¼ cup water and the onion and garlic. Mix well. Cover. Microwave at High for 3½ to 5½ minutes, or until onion is very tender.

Place mixture in blender. Add garbanzo beans. Process until smooth. Cover with plastic wrap. Chill for at least 1 hour before serving. Add water, if desired, for thinner consistency. Garnish with parsley. Serve as dip or spread with crackers or pita bread wedges.

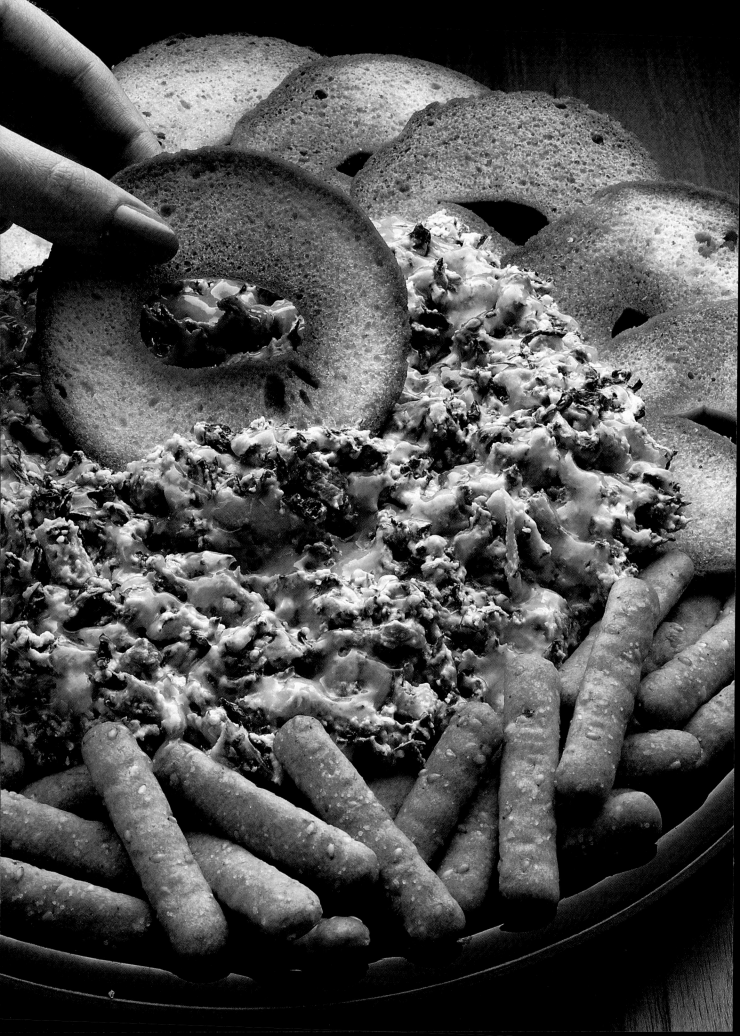

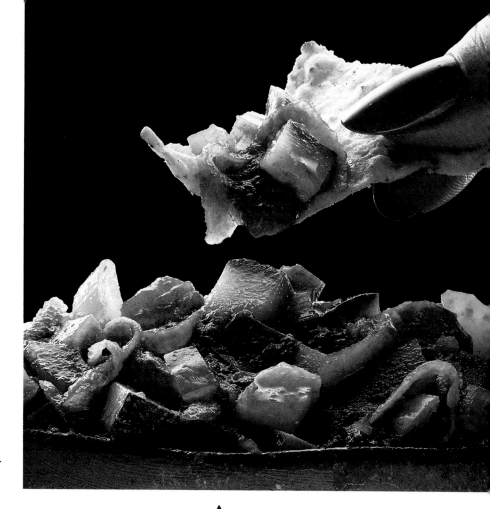

◄ 3-Cheese Spinach Dip

1 cup ricotta cheese
1 pkg. (1.4 oz.) vegetable soup and recipe mix
1 pkg. (10 oz.) frozen chopped spinach
1 pkg. (8 oz.) Neufchâtel cheese
1 jar (2 oz.) sliced pimiento, drained
⅓ cup finely shredded Cheddar cheese
  Bagel chips
  Assorted bread sticks

About 3 cups

In medium mixing bowl, blend ricotta and vegetable soup mix. Cover and chill for 30 minutes to rehydrate dried vegetables. Unwrap spinach and place on plate. Microwave at High for 4 to 6 minutes, or until spinach is defrosted. Drain thoroughly, pressing to remove excess moisture. Add spinach to ricotta mixture. Mix well. Set aside.

Place Neufchâtel on plate. Microwave at 50% (Medium) for 1½ to 3 minutes, or until cheese softens. Add to spinach and ricotta mixture. Add pimiento, and mix well. Spread to 8-inch diameter on 12-inch round platter. Sprinkle with Cheddar cheese. Microwave at 70% (Medium High) for 5 to 7 minutes, or until dip is hot, rotating platter once. Arrange bagel chips and bread sticks around outer edge of platter to serve.

Spicy & Chunky Fresh Dip ▲

2 medium tomatoes, seeded and chopped
1 can (8 oz.) tomato sauce
½ cup chopped zucchini
⅓ cup chopped celery
⅓ cup shredded carrot
¼ cup chopped onion
¼ cup chopped green pepper
½ teaspoon garlic salt
¼ teaspoon sugar
⅛ teaspoon fennel or cumin seed, crushed
2 tablespoons chopped pickled hot peppers

About 2½ cups

In 2-quart casserole, combine all ingredients, except pickled peppers. Cover. Microwave at High for 10 to 13 minutes, or until celery and green pepper are tender-crisp, stirring once. Stir in pickled peppers. Cover and chill for at least 4 hours before serving. Serve dip with tortilla chips.

Gouda Cheese Fondue

1 clove garlic, cut in half
7 oz. Gouda cheese, shredded
2 tablespoons all-purpose flour
  Dash ground nutmeg
  Dash onion powder
½ cup dry white wine
  Cubes of crusty French bread
  Carrot and celery sticks

About 1 cup

Rub inside of 1-quart casserole with cut garlic. Discard garlic. In large plastic food-storage bag, combine cheese, flour, nutmeg and onion powder. Shake to coat cheese. Set aside.

In prepared casserole, microwave wine at 70% (Medium High) for 2 to 3 minutes, or until hot but not boiling. Stir in cheese mixture. Microwave at 70% (Medium High) for 3 to 5 minutes, or until mixture is smooth, stirring vigorously with a whisk 2 or 3 times. Serve hot fondue with bread cubes, carrot and celery sticks.

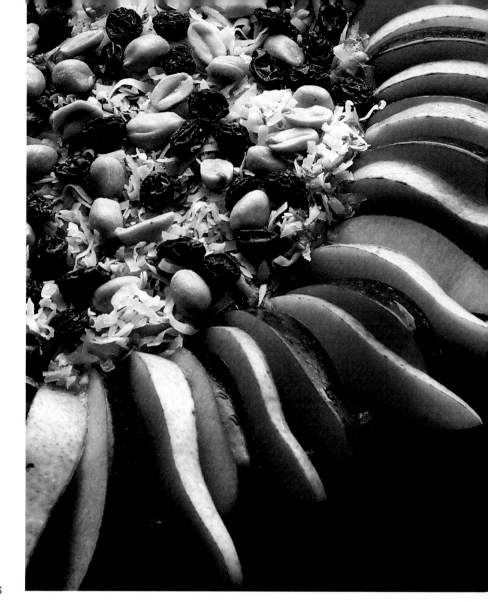

Indian Fruit Dip Platter

1 cup flaked coconut
2 pkgs. (8 oz. each) cream cheese, cut into 1-inch cubes
1 teaspoon grated orange peel
¾ to 1 teaspoon curry powder
⅓ cup chutney
¼ cup raisins
¼ cup salted peanuts
2 pears, cored and cut into ¼-inch slices
2 red apples, cored and cut into ¼-inch slices
2 tablespoons lemon juice
1 tablespoon water

8 to 10 servings

How to Microwave Indian Fruit Dip Platter

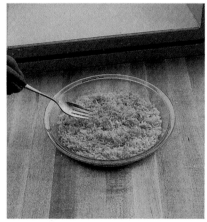

Spread coconut in an even layer in 9-inch pie plate. Microwave at High for 3 to 5 minutes, or just until coconut is golden brown, tossing with fork after every minute. Set aside.

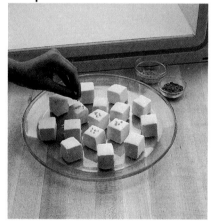

Place cream cheese cubes in an even layer on 12-inch round platter. Sprinkle with orange peel and curry powder. Microwave at 50% (Medium) for 1½ to 3 minutes, or until cream cheese softens. Blend mixture together.

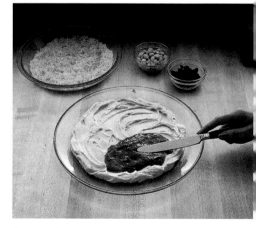

Spread evenly to within 1 or 2 inches from edge of platter. Spread chutney over cream cheese. Top with coconut, raisins and peanuts. Set aside.

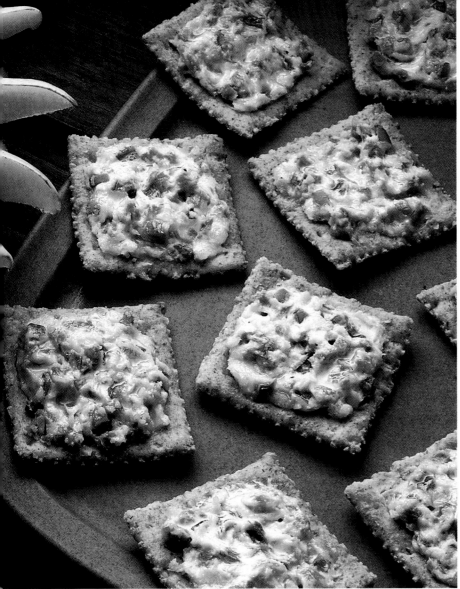

◄ ## Hot Ham-n-Cheese Crackers

> 1 pkg. (3 oz.) cream cheese
> ⅓ cup finely chopped boiled ham
> ⅓ cup shredded Monterey Jack cheese
> 2 tablespoons finely chopped green pepper
> ⅛ teaspoon onion salt
>   Dash pepper
> 24 wheat crackers

2 dozen appetizers

In small mixing bowl, microwave cream cheese at High for 15 to 30 seconds, or until softened. Mix in ham, Monterey Jack cheese, green pepper, onion salt and pepper. Spread about 1 teaspoon of ham and cheese mixture on each cracker. Layer 2 paper towels on plate. Arrange 12 crackers on prepared plate. Microwave at High for 45 seconds to 1½ minutes, or until cheese melts, rotating plate once. Repeat for remaining crackers.

Chopped Chicken Liver Spread

½ lb. chicken livers, rinsed and drained
⅓ cup chopped onion
2 tablespoons snipped fresh parsley
1 tablespoon red wine vinegar
¼ teaspoon dried dill weed

2 hard-cooked eggs, chopped
⅓ cup sour cream
¼ cup mayonnaise
½ teaspoon salt
½ teaspoon Worcestershire sauce
¼ teaspoon pepper

About 1¾ cups

In 1-quart casserole, combine livers, onion, parsley, vinegar and dill weed. Cover. Microwave at 50% (Medium) for 6½ to 9½ minutes, or until livers are no longer pink, stirring once or twice. Cool slightly. Drain.

Chop liver mixture. Place in small mixing bowl. Add remaining ingredients. Mix well. Chill for at least 1 hour before serving. Serve as spread with melba rounds or cocktail bread. Sprinkle with additional snipped fresh parsley, if desired.

Combine fruit, lemon juice and water in medium mixing bowl. Toss to coat fruit. Drain. Arrange fruit slices around outside edge of platter to serve.

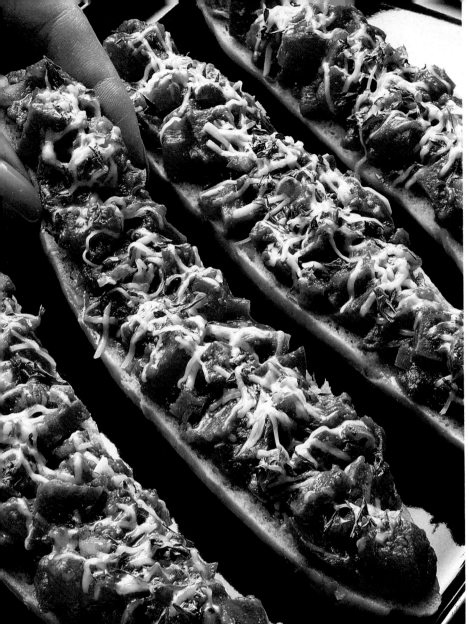

◄ Pizza Bread Sticks

   2 soft bread sticks (6 × 2-inch),
       cut in half lengthwise
   ¼ cup seeded chopped tomato
   ¼ cup finely chopped Canadian
       bacon or pepperoni
   ¼ cup pizza sauce
   1 tablespoon finely chopped
       green pepper
   2 tablespoons shredded
       Parmesan cheese
   ½ teaspoon dried parsley flakes
       Dash garlic powder

4 servings

Arrange bread sticks cut-side-up around edge of paper-towel-lined plate or platter. Set aside. In small mixing bowl, combine tomato, Canadian bacon, pizza sauce and green pepper. Mix well. Spoon evenly over tops of bread sticks. Set aside.

In small bowl, combine remaining ingredients. Sprinkle evenly over bread sticks. Microwave at 70% (Medium High) for 2 to 3 minutes, or until bread sticks are hot, rotating plate once.

Eggplant & Pepper Pita Canapés

   3 cups peeled, cubed
       eggplant (¾-inch cubes)
   1 tablespoon vegetable oil
   1 tablespoon vinegar
   ½ teaspoon Italian seasoning
   1 clove garlic, minced
   ¼ cup chopped red pepper
   2 tablespoons mayonnaise or
       sour cream
   1 tablespoon snipped fresh
       parsley
   ¼ teaspoon salt
   2 whole wheat pita breads
       (6-inch)
  16 sliced pimiento-stuffed green
       olives

16 appetizers

In 1-quart casserole, combine eggplant, oil, vinegar, Italian seasoning and garlic. Cover. Microwave at High for 7 to 10 minutes, or until eggplant is very tender, stirring once. Place eggplant mixture in food processor or blender. Process until smooth. Return mixture to casserole. Add red pepper, mayonnaise, parsley and salt. Mix well.

To serve, arrange pita breads on baking sheet. Place under conventional broiler. Broil 3 inches from heat until breads are toasted, about 4 minutes, turning over once. Cut each pita bread into quarters, then split each quarter into 2 wedges. Spread each wedge with about 1 tablespoon of filling and top with a sliced olive.

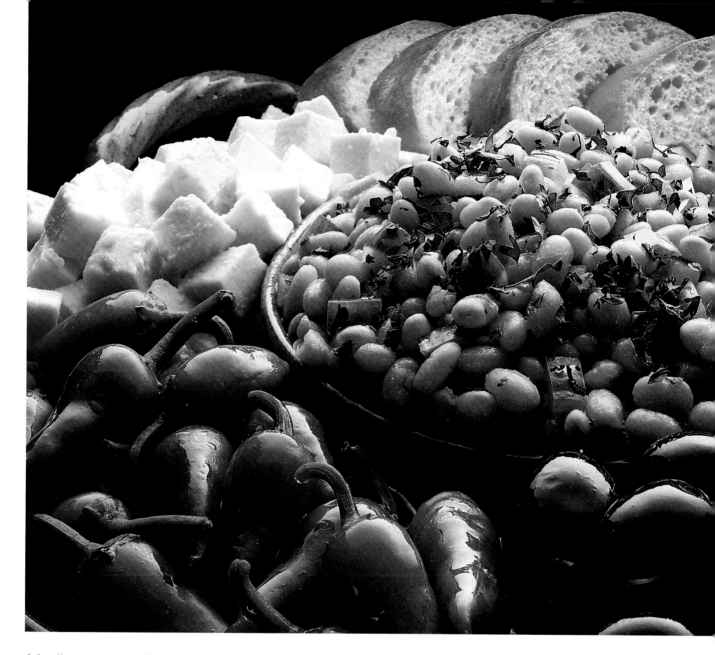

Mediterranean Snack Platter

1½ cups dried navy beans
1 quart hot water
1 small onion, cut into quarters
¼ teaspoon dried thyme leaves
½ cup chopped red onion
½ cup olive oil
¼ cup red wine vinegar
2 teaspoons dried parsley flakes
1 teaspoon dried oregano leaves
1 teaspoon salt
¼ teaspoon pepper
  Greek olives
  Hot peppers
  Feta cheese

Sort, rinse and drain beans. In 3-quart casserole, combine beans, water, onion quarters and thyme. Cover. Microwave at High for 8 to 12 minutes, or until water boils. Microwave at 50% (Medium) for 1 to 1¾ hours, or just until beans are tender, stirring 2 or 3 times. Drain beans. Discard liquid and onion. In medium mixing bowl, place beans and red onion. Set aside.

In small bowl, blend olive oil, vinegar, parsley, oregano, salt and pepper. Pour mixture over beans. Mix well. Cover with plastic wrap. Refrigerate for at least 8 hours, or overnight.

To serve: Microwave beans at High for 1 to 2½ minutes, or until warm, stirring once. Using slotted spoon, arrange one-half the beans on serving platter with Greek olives, hot peppers and feta cheese. Garnish with snipped fresh parsley and serve with thin slices French bread, if desired. Replenish platter with remaining beans.

2 platters (8 to 10 servings each)

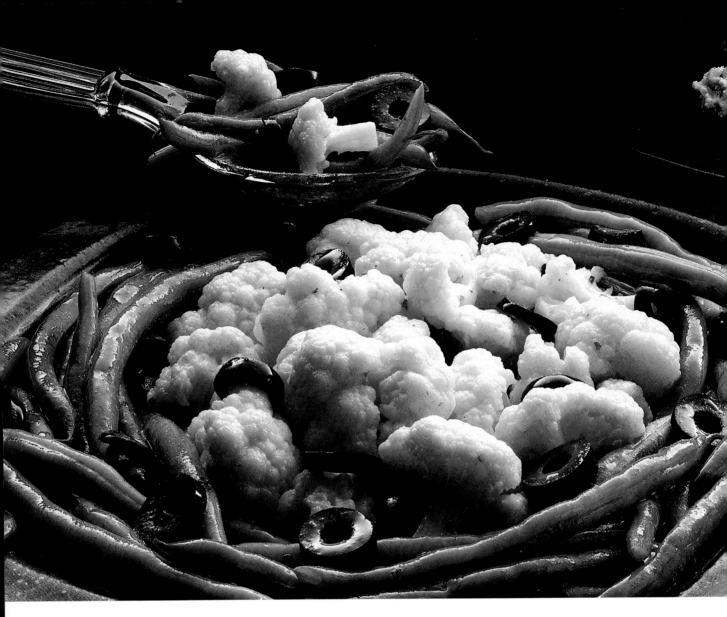

Marinated Vegetable Arrangement

2 cups fresh cauliflowerets
8 oz. fresh whole green beans, trimmed
2 tablespoons water
1 tablespoon vinegar
¼ teaspoon dried marjoram leaves
2 tablespoons sliced black olives

Dressing:

⅓ cup vegetable oil
1 tablespoon vinegar
2 teaspoons Dijon mustard
¼ teaspoon salt
¼ teaspoon dried marjoram leaves
Dash pepper

6 to 8 servings

How to Microwave a Marinated Vegetable Arrangement

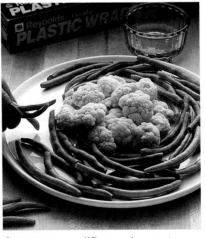

Arrange cauliflower in center of 12-inch round platter. Place green beans around cauliflower. In small dish, combine water and vinegar. Pour over vegetables.

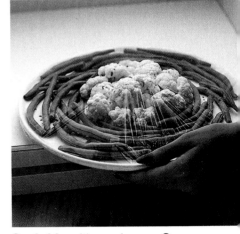

Sprinkle with marjoram. Cover platter with plastic wrap. Microwave at High for 8 to 13 minutes, or until beans are tender-crisp, rotating platter once. Drain. Add olives to platter. Set aside.

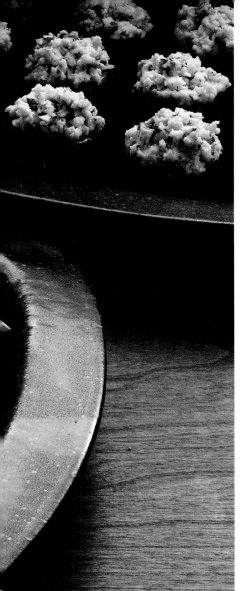

◀ Pesto & Cheese Tomatoes

1 pint cherry tomatoes	2 tablespoons grated Parmesan cheese
1 tablespoon finely chopped onion	2 tablespoons pesto*
1 teaspoon olive oil	1 tablespoon snipped fresh parsley
⅔ cup ricotta cheese	

2 dozen appetizers

Cut thin slice from stem end of each tomato. With small spoon or melon baller, scoop out pulp. Discard pulp and tops of tomatoes. Place tomatoes cut-side-down on paper towel to drain.

In small mixing bowl, combine onion and olive oil. Microwave at High for 30 seconds to 1 minute, or until onion is tender. Stir in remaining ingredients. Stuff tomatoes with cheese mixture. Arrange tomatoes on paper-towel-lined plate, with smaller tomatoes in the center. Microwave at High for 1 to 2 minutes, or until mixture is hot, rotating plate once.

*Pesto is available in gourmet section of supermarkets.

Cocktail Snacks ▶

Marinade:
- ⅓ cup gin
- 2 tablespoons fresh lemon juice
- 1 tablespoon vegetable oil
- ¼ teaspoon dried basil leaves
- ⅛ teaspoon garlic salt
- 2 slices lemon
- 2 whole allspice

- 12 whole small fresh mushrooms (1-inch)
- 12 pimiento-stuffed green olives
- 12 small boiled whole onions

12 appetizers

In 1-quart casserole, combine all marinade ingredients. Add mushrooms. Cover. Microwave at High for 2 to 3 minutes, or until mushrooms are very hot, stirring once. Stir in olives and onions. Re-cover. Chill for at least 3 hours. Drain marinade and discard lemon slices and allspice.

On each of 12 cocktail picks, skewer an onion, olive and mushroom. Arrange on serving plate. Or use as garnish for gin or vodka-based drinks.

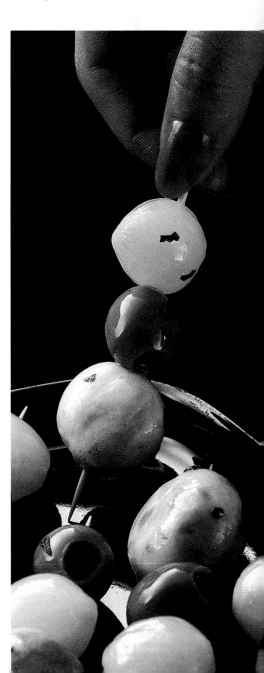

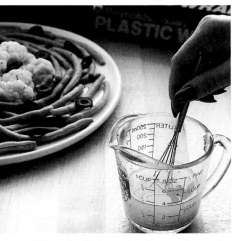

Blend all dressing ingredients in 1-cup measure. Pour evenly over vegetables. Re-cover with plastic wrap. Chill for at least 3 hours before serving.

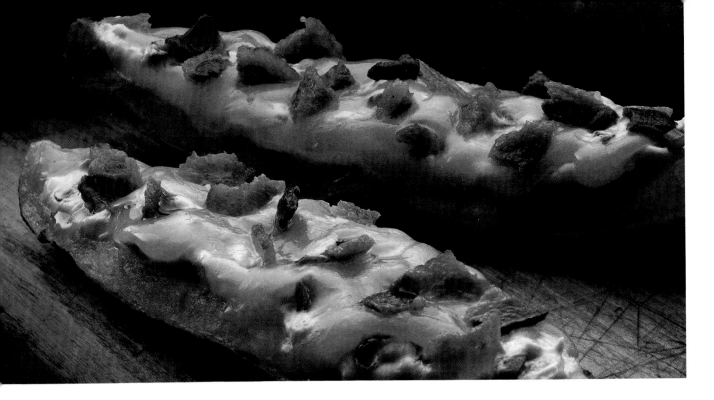

Cheesy Bacon Skins

4 slices bacon
¼ cup sour cream
1 tablespoon sliced green onion
1 teaspoon prepared horseradish
8 Potato Skins (below)
½ cup shredded Cheddar cheese

4 servings

Layer 3 paper towels on a plate. Arrange bacon slices on paper towels and cover with another paper towel. Microwave bacon at High for 3 to 6 minutes, or until brown and crisp. Cool and crumble. Set aside.

In small bowl, combine sour cream, onion and horseradish. Mix well. Divide mixture into 8 equal portions. Spread 1 portion onto each potato skin. Sprinkle skins evenly with crumbled bacon and shredded cheese. Microwave at 50% (Medium) for 3½ to 7 minutes, or until skins are hot and cheese is melted, rotating plate once. Serve with additional sour cream, if desired.

How to Prepare Potato Skins

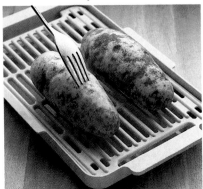

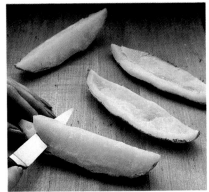

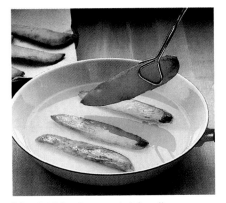

Pierce 2 baking potatoes (8 to 10 oz. each) with fork. Arrange on roasting rack, or wrap each potato in paper towel. Microwave at High for 5 to 10 minutes, or until potatoes are tender, turning over and rearranging once. Let stand for 10 minutes.

Cut each potato lengthwise into 4 equal wedges. Carefully cut center away from each wedge, leaving ¼-inch shell. Reserve centers for use in other recipes.

Heat ½ inch vegetable oil conventionally in deep 10-inch skillet over medium-high heat. Fry potato skins until deep golden brown, 8 to 10 minutes. Drain on paper towels. Arrange potato skins cut-side-up on paper-towel-lined plate. Set aside.

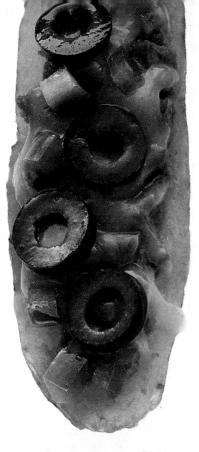

Pizza Potato Skins ▲

¼ cup pizza sauce
¼ cup finely chopped pepperoni
1 tablespoon finely chopped onion
1 tablespoon finely chopped green pepper (optional)
8 Potato Skins (opposite)
½ cup shredded mozzarella cheese

Toppings:
Chopped tomato
Chopped green pepper
Sliced black or pimiento-stuffed green olives
Sour cream

4 servings

In small bowl, combine pizza sauce, pepperoni, onion and green pepper. Mix well. Divide mixture into 8 equal portions. Spread 1 portion onto each potato skin. Sprinkle skins evenly with cheese. Microwave at 50% (Medium) for 3½ to 7 minutes, or until skins are hot and cheese is melted, rotating plate once. Before serving, add one or more of the toppings.

Cream Cheese & Shrimp-topped Skins ▼

1 pkg. (3 oz.) cream cheese
1 can (4¼ oz.) small shrimp, rinsed and drained
⅛ teaspoon cayenne
8 Potato Skins (opposite)
¼ cup shredded Cheddar cheese
¼ cup shredded Monterey Jack cheese
2 tablespoons sliced green onion or chopped green pepper
Lemon wedges
Cocktail sauce

4 servings

In small mixing bowl, microwave cream cheese at High for 15 to 30 seconds, or until softened. Stir. Gently mix in shrimp and cayenne. Divide mixture into 8 equal portions. Spread 1 portion onto each potato skin. Sprinkle skins evenly with cheeses and onion. Microwave at 50% (Medium) for 3½ to 7 minutes, or until skins are hot and cheeses are melted, rotating plate once. Serve with lemon wedges and cocktail sauce.

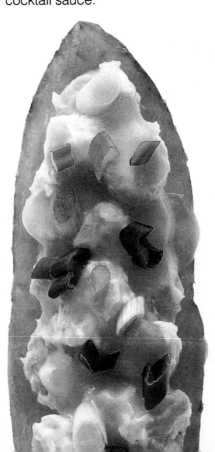

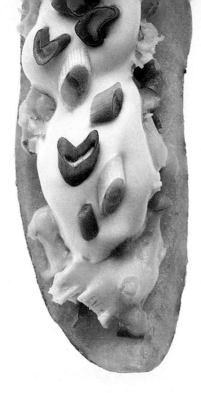

Herb Chicken Potato Skins ▲

1 can (5 oz.) chunk chicken, drained
2 tablespoons Italian dressing
2 tablespoons grated Parmesan cheese
2 tablespoons finely chopped green pepper (optional)
¼ teaspoon dried marjoram leaves
⅛ teaspoon garlic powder
⅛ teaspoon pepper
8 Potato Skins (opposite)
½ cup shredded Monterey Jack cheese
Sour cream
Sliced green onions

4 servings

In small mixing bowl, combine chicken, Italian dressing, Parmesan cheese, green pepper, marjoram, garlic and pepper. Mix well. Divide mixture into 8 equal portions. Spread 1 portion onto each potato skin. Sprinkle skins evenly with Monterey Jack cheese. Microwave at 50% (Medium) for 3½ to 7 minutes, or until skins are hot and cheese is melted, rotating plate once. Before serving, top with sour cream and green onions.

Snack Pizza Crusts

Yellow cornmeal
1 can (11 oz.) refrigerated soft
    bread sticks

1 tablespoon olive oil
⅛ teaspoon garlic powder

Dried Italian seasoning
    (optional)

4 snack crusts

How to Bake Snack Pizza Crusts

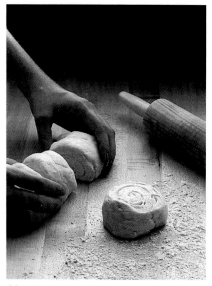

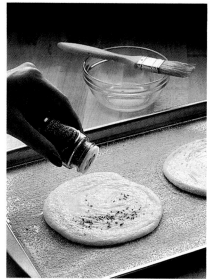

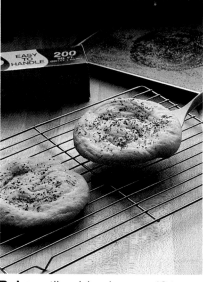

Heat conventional oven to 400°F. Grease 2 baking sheets with shortening. Sprinkle lightly with cornmeal. Set aside. Separate dough into 4 portions. Place cut-side-up on floured board. With rolling pin, firmly roll one portion at a time to 6-inch diameter.

Place 2 rounds of dough on each prepared baking sheet. Prick each round several times with fork. In small bowl, combine oil and garlic powder. Brush oil mixture lightly onto each dough surface. Sprinkle each lightly with Italian seasoning.

Bake until golden brown, 12 to 15 minutes, switching baking sheets on racks after half the time. Remove to cooling rack and cool completely. Wrap and store at room temperature for no longer than 2 days. Or wrap and freeze for no longer than 1 month.

How to Defrost Snack Pizza Crusts

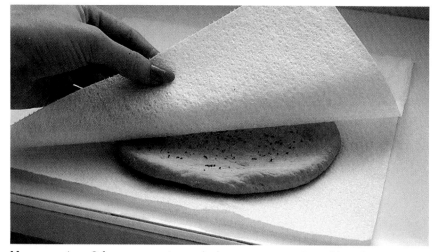

Unwrap 1 or 2 frozen crusts and place on paper towel in microwave. Cover with another paper towel. Microwave 1 crust at High for 20 to 30 seconds, or until defrosted. Microwave 2 crusts at High for 40 to 55 seconds, or until defrosted.

Pizza Sauce

1 can (16 oz.) whole tomatoes, drained and chopped
3 tablespoons tomato paste
½ teaspoon dried parsley flakes
½ teaspoon dried basil leaves
¼ teaspoon dried oregano leaves
¼ teaspoon sugar
⅛ to ¼ teaspoon crushed red pepper flakes

About 1 cup

In 1-quart casserole, combine all ingredients. Microwave, uncovered, at High for 7½ to 15 minutes, or until sauce is very thick and flavors are blended, stirring 2 or 3 times. Store in refrigerator for no longer than one week.

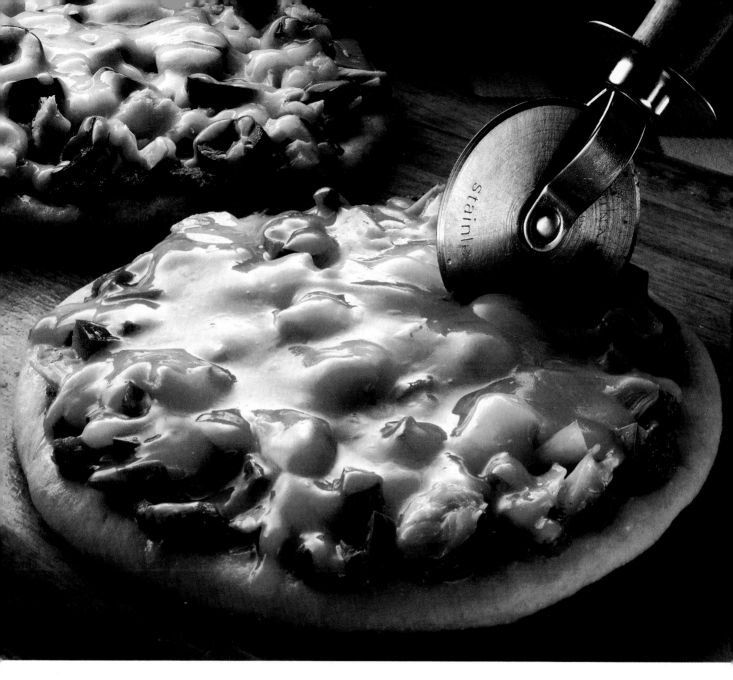

Tuna & Olive Pizza ▲

- 1 Snack Pizza Crust (opposite)
- ¼ cup Pizza Sauce (opposite)
- ¼ cup drained and flaked canned tuna
- 1 tablespoon sliced black olives
- ¼ cup shredded Swiss cheese

1 serving

Spread crust with sauce. Top evenly with tuna and olives. Sprinkle with cheese. Place on paper-towel-lined plate. Microwave at 70% (Medium High) for 1¾ to 3¼ minutes, or until cheese melts, rotating plate once.

Artichoke & Pepper Pizza ▲

- 1 Snack Pizza Crust (opposite)
- ¼ cup Pizza Sauce (opposite)
- 3 marinated artichoke hearts, drained and chopped
- 1 tablespoon chopped red pepper
- 2 tablespoons shredded Cheddar cheese
- 2 tablespoons shredded Monterey Jack cheese

1 serving

Spread crust with sauce. Top evenly with artichoke hearts and red pepper. Sprinkle with cheeses. Place on paper-towel-lined plate. Microwave at 70% (Medium High) for 1¾ to 3¼ minutes, or until cheeses melt, rotating plate once.

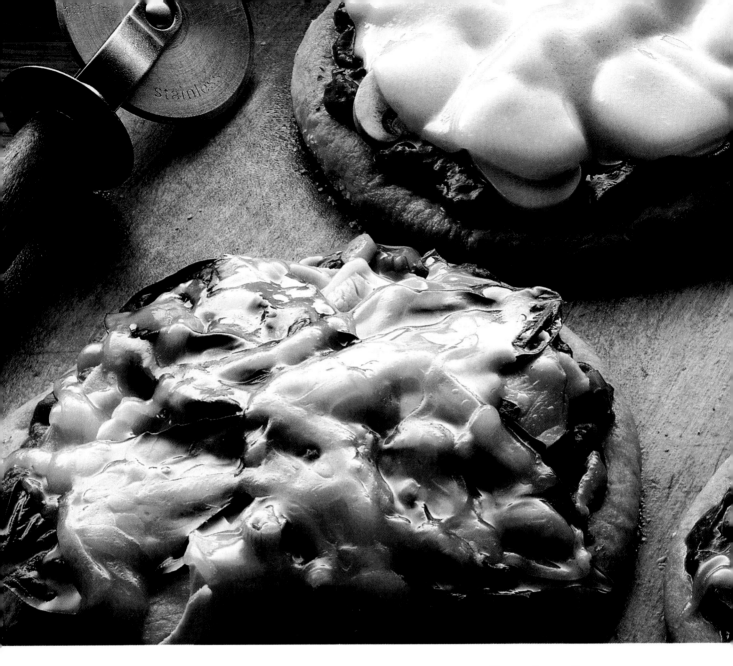

Turkey & Fresh Basil Pizza ▲

1 Snack Pizza Crust (page 20)
¼ cup Pizza Sauce (page 20)
1 thin slice (1 oz.) fully cooked
  turkey breast
1 green onion, thinly sliced

4 large fresh basil leaves
2 tablespoons shredded Colby
  cheese
2 tablespoons shredded Swiss
  cheese

1 serving

Spread crust with sauce. Top with turkey slice, green onion and basil leaves. Sprinkle with cheeses. Place on paper-towel-lined plate. Microwave at 70% (Medium High) for 1¾ to 3¼ minutes, or until cheeses melt, rotating plate once.

Prosciutto & ▲
Mushroom Pizza

1 Snack Pizza Crust (page 20)
¼ cup Pizza Sauce (page 20)
1 oz. shaved Prosciutto or
  boiled ham
2 tablespoons sliced fresh or
  canned mushrooms
1 slice (1 oz.) Provolone cheese

1 serving

Spread crust with sauce. Top with Prosciutto and mushrooms. Add cheese. Place on paper-towel-lined plate. Microwave at 70% (Medium High) for 1¾ to 3¼ minutes, or until cheese melts, rotating plate once.

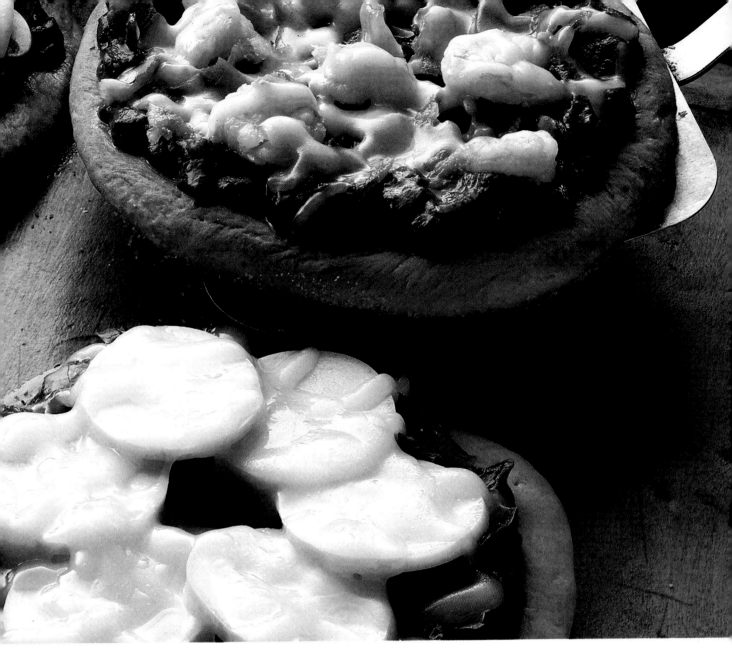

Summertime Pizza ▲

1 Snack Pizza Crust (page 20)
¼ cup Pizza Sauce (page 20)
½ cup loosely packed, torn fresh spinach leaves
6 thin slices yellow summer squash
¼ cup shredded mozzarella cheese

1 serving

Spread crust with sauce. Top with spinach and summer squash slices. Sprinkle with cheese. Place on paper-towel-lined plate. Microwave at 70% (Medium High) for 1¾ to 3¼ minutes, or until cheese melts, rotating plate once.

Shrimp & Bacon Pizza ▲

1 Snack Pizza Crust (page 20)
¼ cup Pizza Sauce (page 20)
2 slices bacon
¼ cup canned medium shrimp, rinsed and drained
¼ cup shredded Muenster cheese

1 serving

Spread crust with sauce. Set aside. Place bacon on roasting rack. Cover with paper towel. Microwave at High for 1½ to 2½ minutes, or until brown and crisp. Cool slightly and crumble. Top pizza with bacon and shrimp. Sprinkle with cheese. Place on paper-towel-lined plate. Microwave at 70% (Medium High) for 1¾ to 3¼ minutes, or until cheese melts, rotating plate once.

Clam & Bacon Pizza: Follow recipe above, except substitute 2 tablespoons canned drained clams for shrimp.

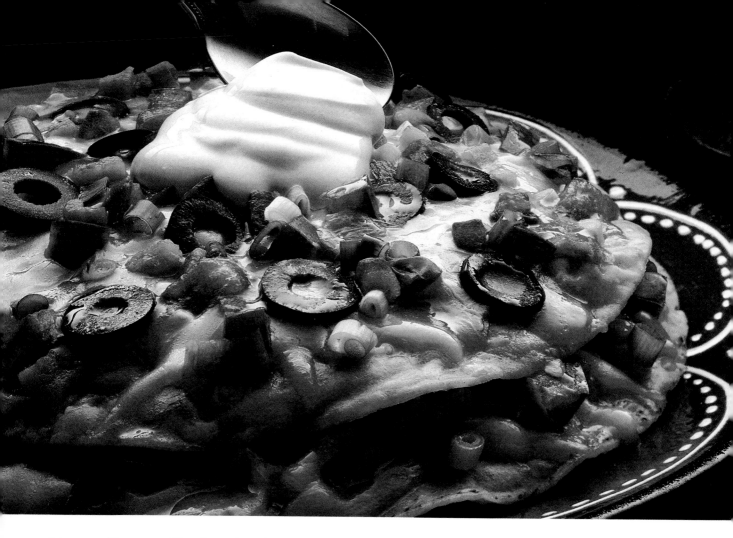

How to Prepare Tortillas for Cheese Crisps

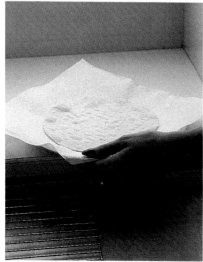

Microwave: Place one 8-inch flour tortilla on paper-towel-lined plate. Microwave at High for 1¾ to 2¼ minutes, or just until surface is dry and puffy, rotating plate once. Remove tortilla to cooling rack to cool and crisp. Repeat for additional tortillas.

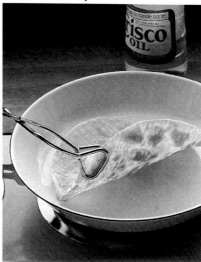

Conventional: Heat 2 tablespoons oil in 10-inch skillet over medium-high heat. Add one 8-inch flour tortilla and fry until golden brown. Turn and fry other side. Drain tortilla on paper towels. Repeat for additional tortillas. Add additional oil during frying, if necessary.

South of the Border Cheese Crisp

  2 prepared tortillas (left)
  1 cup shredded Colby cheese
  ½ cup shredded mozzarella cheese
  ½ cup seeded chopped tomato
  2 tablespoons sliced black olives
  2 tablespoons sliced green onion
  2 tablespoons chopped green chilies, drained
     Sour cream

4 to 6 servings

Place 1 tortilla on 10-inch plate. Top with half of the cheeses, tomato, olives, green onion and chilies. Top with remaining tortilla and remaining ingredients, except sour cream. Microwave at High for 2 to 2½ minutes, or until cheeses melt, rotating plate once or twice. Top with sour cream. Cut into wedges to serve.

Fresh Vegetable Cheese Crisp

- 1 pkg. (3 oz.) cream cheese
- ¼ cup plus 2 tablespoons sharp Cheddar cheese, divided
- ½ teaspoon dried basil leaves Dash garlic powder
- 2 prepared tortillas (opposite)
- 1 cup fresh broccoli flowerets
- 1 tablespoon water
- ½ cup sliced fresh mushrooms
- 3 thin red pepper rings

4 to 6 servings

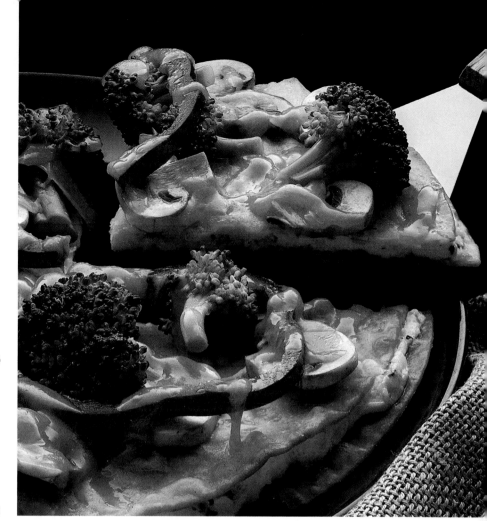

How to Microwave Fresh Vegetable Cheese Crisp

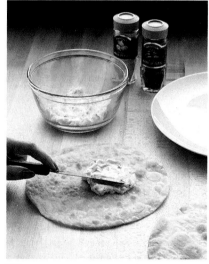

Microwave cream cheese in small bowl at High for 15 to 30 seconds, or until softened. Stir in 2 tablespoons Cheddar cheese, the basil and garlic powder. Spread on 1 tortilla. Top with remaining tortilla. Place on plate. Set aside.

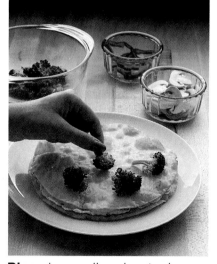

Place broccoli and water in 1-quart casserole. Cover. Microwave at High for 1 to 2 minutes, or until broccoli is tender-crisp. Drain. Arrange broccoli, mushrooms and red pepper on cheese crisp.

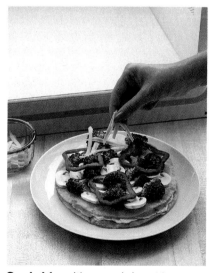

Sprinkle with remaining ¼ cup Cheddar cheese. Microwave at 70% (Medium High) for 2½ to 3½ minutes, or until cheese melts, rotating plate once or twice. Cut into wedges to serve.

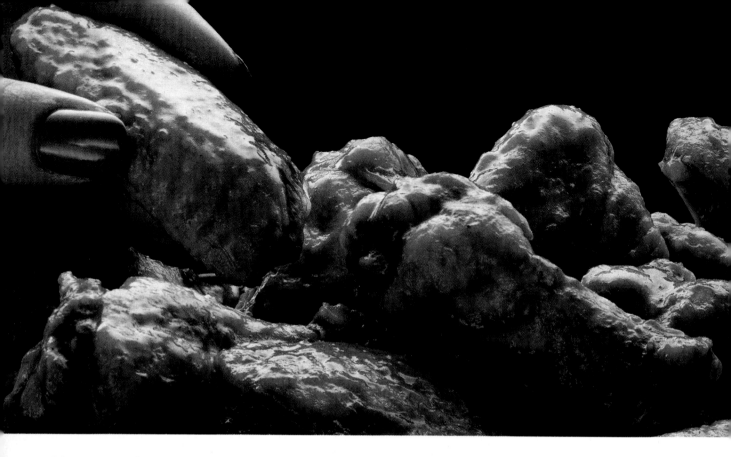

Marinated Chicken Wings

1½ lbs. chicken wings

1 recipe Spicy Sesame, Orange Barbecue, or Hot Garlic Marinade (opposite)

Dipping Sauce (opposite, optional)

6 servings

How to Microwave Marinated Chicken Wings

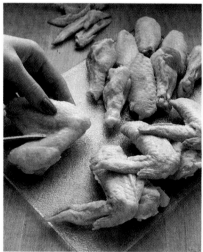

Separate each chicken wing into 3 parts, cutting at joints. Discard wing tips. Set chicken pieces aside.

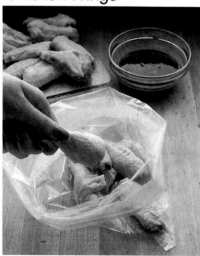

Combine wings and marinade in large plastic food-storage bag. Secure the bag. Refrigerate for at least 2 hours, or overnight, turning once or twice.

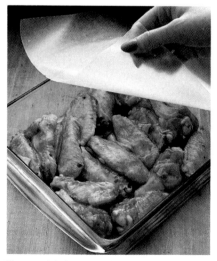

Pour chicken and marinade into 9-inch square baking dish. Cover with wax paper. Microwave at High for 11 to 13 minutes, or until chicken is no longer pink, stirring once or twice. Serve with Dipping Sauce.

Spicy Sesame Marinade

- 2 tablespoons soy sauce
- 2 tablespoons sliced green onion
- 1 tablespoon packed brown sugar
- 1 tablespoon vegetable oil
- 1 teaspoon paprika
- 1 teaspoon sesame oil
- ½ teaspoon celery salt
- ¼ teaspoon crushed red pepper flakes

In 2-cup measure, combine all ingredients. Microwave at High for 1 to 1½ minutes, or until sauce is hot, stirring once. Let marinade cool slightly.

Orange Barbecue Marinade

- ¼ cup barbecue sauce
- 2 tablespoons orange marmalade
- 2 tablespoons orange juice
- 1 teaspoon grated orange peel
- ½ teaspoon onion salt
- ¼ teaspoon curry powder
- ¼ teaspoon crushed red pepper flakes

In small mixing bowl, combine all ingredients. Mix well.

Hot Garlic Marinade

- ¼ cup steak sauce
- ¼ cup catsup
- 2 cloves garlic, minced
- ½ teaspoon chili powder
- ¼ teaspoon cayenne

In 2-cup measure, combine all ingredients. Microwave at High for 1 to 1½ minutes, or until sauce is hot, stirring once. Let marinade cool slightly.

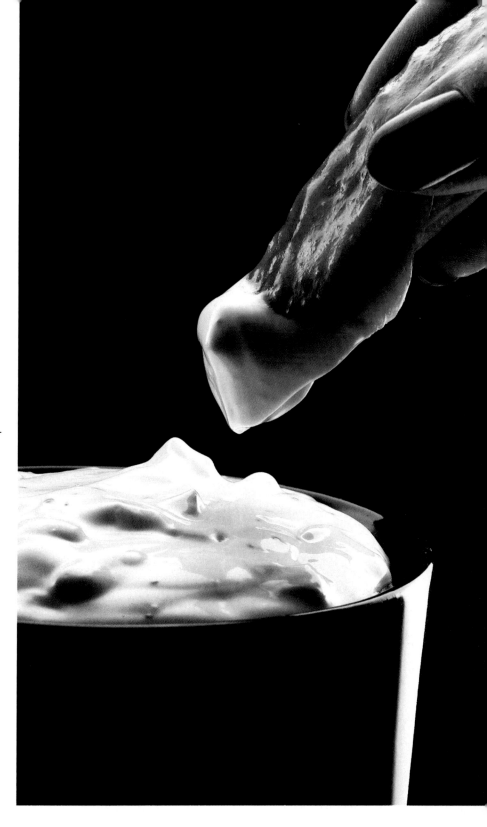

Dipping Sauce ▲

- ¼ cup finely chopped celery
- ¼ cup mayonnaise
- 3 tablespoons sour cream
- ⅛ teaspoon celery salt
- Dash garlic powder

About ½ cup

In small bowl, combine all ingredients. Mix well. Serve with Marinated Chicken Wings (opposite).

27

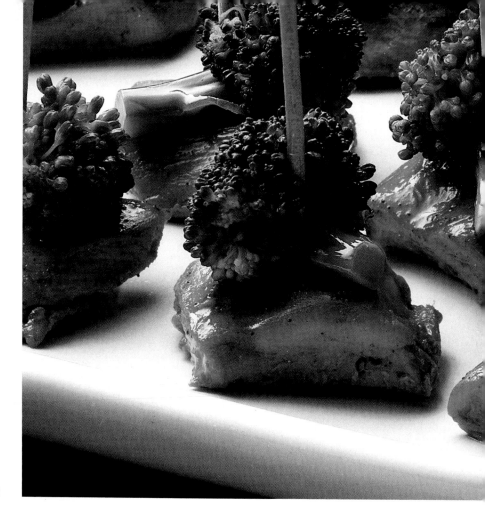

Chicken & Broccoli Bites

- 1 boneless whole chicken breast (about 12 oz.)
- ⅓ cup teriyaki sauce
- 1 tablespoon vegetable oil
- ½ teaspoon grated orange peel
- ⅛ teaspoon ground cinnamon
- ⅛ teaspoon ground coriander
- ⅛ teaspoon pepper
- 12 oz. fresh broccoli

4 servings

How to Microwave Chicken & Broccoli Bites

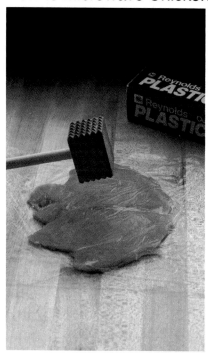

Remove and discard chicken skin. Pound chicken breast between 2 sheets of plastic wrap to about ¼-inch thickness. Cut into about 1¼-inch square pieces.

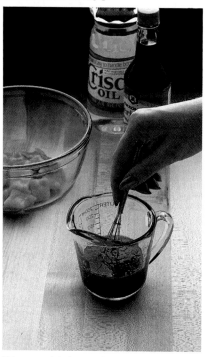

Place chicken pieces in small mixing bowl. Set aside. In 1-cup measure, combine teriyaki, oil, orange peel, cinnamon, coriander and pepper. Mix well.

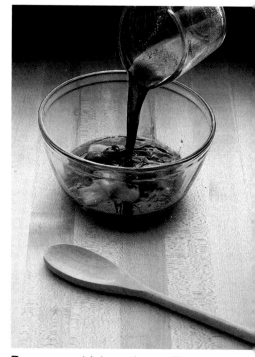

Pour over chicken pieces. Toss to coat. Cover and refrigerate for at least 2 hours. Drain chicken, discarding marinade.

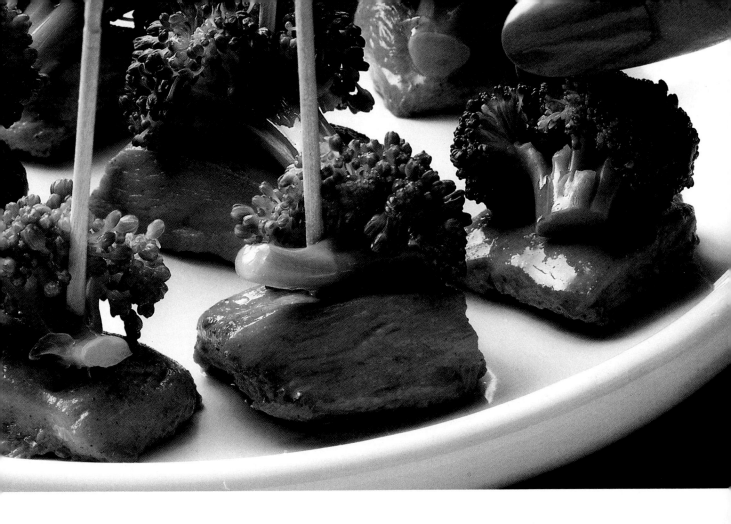

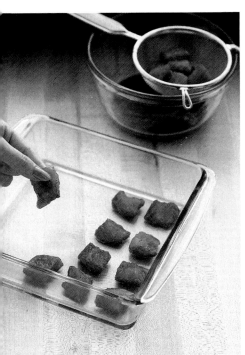

Arrange chicken pieces in single layer in 9-inch square baking dish. Set aside. Cut broccoli into flowerets. Reserve stalk for future use in other recipes.

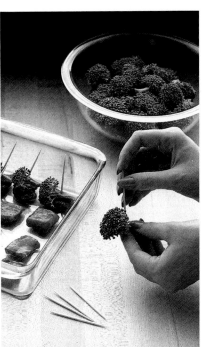

Skewer 1 broccoli floweret with wooden pick. Place pick into chicken piece so broccoli portion is on top. Picks will stand upright.

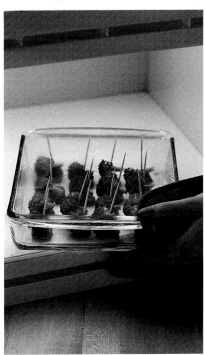

Cover dish with plastic wrap. Microwave at High for 4½ to 6 minutes, or until chicken is firm and no longer pink and broccoli is tender-crisp, rearranging once.

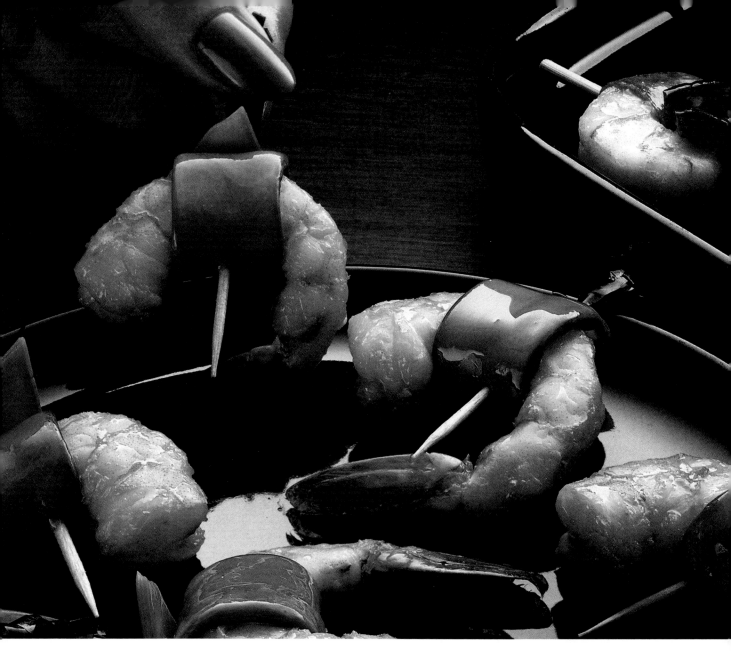

Pea-Pod-wrapped Shrimp ▲ How to Microwave Pea-Pod-wrapped Shrimp

12 fresh pea pods, 3½ inches or
    longer
12 medium shrimp, shelled and
    deveined
 3 tablespoons soy sauce
 1 tablespoon vegetable oil
 2 teaspoons lime juice
¼ teaspoon chili powder
¼ teaspoon ground ginger
 1 clove garlic, minced

12 appetizers

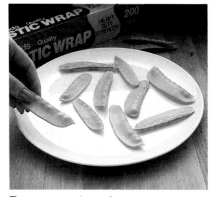

Remove strings from pea pods. Arrange pods on plate. Sprinkle with water. Cover with plastic wrap. Microwave at High for 1 to 1½ minutes, or just until pea pods are flexible. Cool slightly.

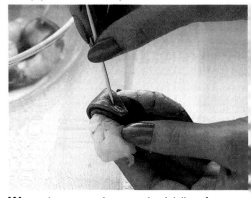

Wrap 1 pea pod around middle of each shrimp. Secure with wooden pick. Place wrapped shrimp in 9-inch round cake dish. Set aside.

30

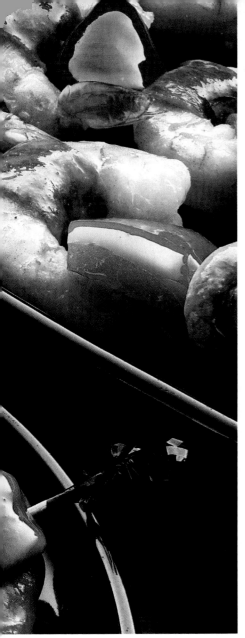

Shrimp & Pepper Kabobs

- 4 thin slices hard salami
- 12 medium shrimp, shelled and deveined
- 6 wooden skewers (6-inch)
- ½ small red pepper, cut into 6 chunks
- ½ small green pepper, cut into 6 chunks
- 6 fresh mushrooms
- 2 tablespoons butter or margarine
- ¼ teaspoon onion powder
- ⅛ teaspoon dry mustard
  Dash dried thyme leaves

6 kabobs

Cut each slice of salami into 3 equal strips. Wrap 1 salami strip around middle of each shrimp. On each of 6 wooden skewers, thread a salami-wrapped shrimp, a red pepper chunk, another wrapped shrimp, a green pepper chunk and a mushroom. Place on roasting rack. Set aside.

In 1-cup measure, place remaining ingredients. Microwave at High for 45 seconds to 1 minute, or until butter melts. Stir. Brush on kabobs. Microwave at High for 3½ to 5 minutes, or until shrimp are opaque, rearranging kabobs and brushing with butter mixture once.

Shrimp Cocktail

- 1 pkg. (12 oz.) frozen uncooked large shrimp
- ¼ teaspoon dried dill weed
- ⅛ teaspoon pepper
- 1½ cups alfalfa sprouts
- ½ cup sliced celery
- 2 tablespoons chopped onion
- ¾ cup cocktail sauce
- ¼ cup plus 2 tablespoons chopped avocado
  Fresh lemon wedges (optional)

6 servings

Place shrimp in 1½-quart casserole. Sprinkle with dill weed and pepper. Cover. Microwave at 70% (Medium High) for 9 to 15 minutes, or until shrimp are opaque, stirring 2 or 3 times. Drain. Chill for at least 3 hours.

In each of 6 small (6 to 8 oz.) narrow glass bowls, evenly layer the sprouts, celery and onion. Divide shrimp among the 6 bowls, hanging shrimp over edges of bowls with tails facing inside. Spoon cocktail sauce over sprout mixture. Top with avocado. Serve with fresh lemon wedge.

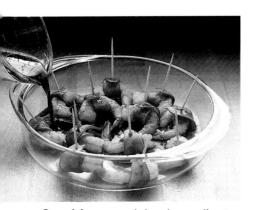

Combine remaining ingredients in 1-cup measure. Mix well. Pour over shrimp. Stir gently to coat. Cover with plastic wrap. Let stand at room temperature for 15 minutes.

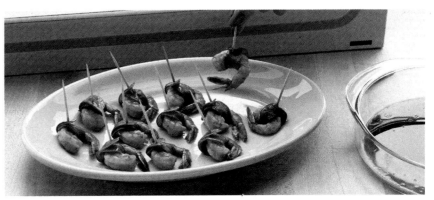

Remove shrimp from marinade and arrange on platter or plate. Discard marinade. Microwave shrimp at 70% (Medium High) for 4 to 5½ minutes, or until shrimp are opaque, rotating platter once or twice.

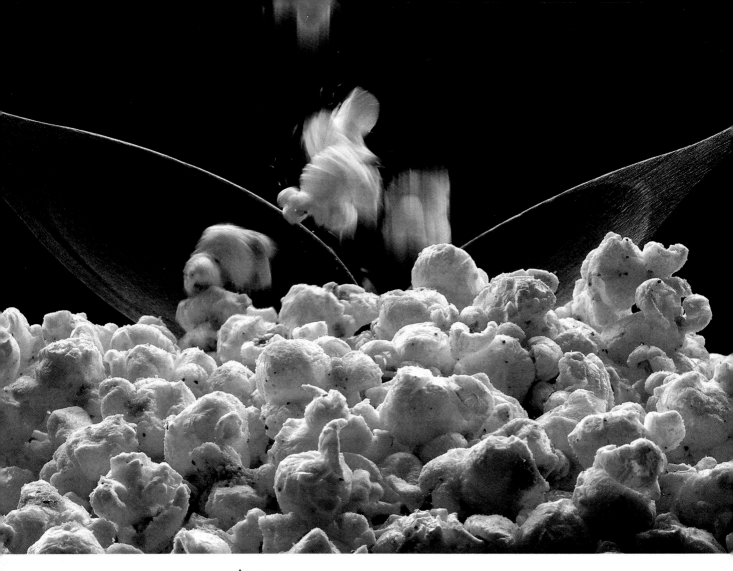

Cheesy Mexican Popcorn

- 8 cups popped popcorn
- ¼ cup plus 2 tablespoons butter or margarine
- 1 teaspoon chili powder
- ¼ teaspoon seasoned salt
- ¼ teaspoon ground cumin
- ⅛ teaspoon cayenne
- ½ cup grated American cheese food

8 cups

Place popcorn in large bowl. Set aside. Place butter in 2-cup measure. Add chili power, seasoned salt, cumin and cayenne. Microwave at High for 1½ to 1¾ minutes, or until butter melts. Stir in cheese. Spoon evenly over popcorn. Using 2 large spoons, toss until popcorn is evenly coated with cheese mixture.

Sour Cream Chive Popcorn

- 8 cups popped popcorn
- ¼ cup butter or margarine
- 1½ teaspoons freeze-dried chives
- 2 tablespoons sour cream sauce mix*

8 cups

Place popcorn in large bowl. Set aside. Place butter in 2-cup measure. Add chives. Microwave at High for 1¼ to 1½ minutes, or until butter melts. Stir in sour cream sauce mix. Spoon evenly over popcorn. Using 2 large spoons, toss until popcorn is evenly coated with butter mixture.

*Half of 1 envelope (1.25 oz.). Save remaining half of envelope for another recipe of Sour Cream Chive Popcorn.

Herb Parmesan Popcorn

- 8 cups popped popcorn
- ¼ cup plus 2 tablespoons butter or margarine
- ½ teaspoon Italian seasoning
- ¼ teaspoon garlic salt
- ½ cup grated Parmesan cheese

8 cups

Place popcorn in large bowl. Set aside. Place butter in 2-cup measure. Add Italian seasoning and garlic salt. Microwave at High for 1½ to 1¾ minutes, or until butter melts. Stir in cheese. Spoon evenly over popcorn. Using 2 large spoons, toss until popcorn is evenly coated with seasoned cheese mixture.

Crunchy Snack Mix ▶

½ cup butter or margarine
1 package (.4 oz.) ranch salad
   dressing mix, buttermilk
   recipe
3 cups oyster crackers
1 can (12 oz.) mixed nuts
2 cups small pretzel twists

7 to 8 cups

In large mixing bowl, microwave
butter at High for 1½ to 1¾ minutes, or until butter melts. Stir in
salad dressing mix. Add remaining ingredients. Toss to coat.
Microwave at High for 4 to 6 minutes, or until mixture is very hot
and butter is absorbed, stirring
once. Spread on paper-towel-
lined baking sheet. Cool completely. Store in covered container.

Seasoned Sticks & Stones

1 can (9 oz.) shoestring
   potatoes
1 cup dry roasted peanuts
⅓ cup butter or margarine
2 teaspoons dried parsley
   flakes
1½ teaspoons chili powder
¼ teaspoon garlic powder
¼ teaspoon cayenne

8 cups

In large bowl, combine shoestring potatoes and peanuts. Set
aside. In 1-cup measure, microwave butter and seasonings at
High for 1½ to 1¾ minutes, or
until butter melts. Mix well. Pour
melted butter mixture over shoestring potatoes and peanuts.
Toss to coat. Microwave at High
for 4 to 6 minutes, or until shoestring potatoes are hot, tossing
with two forks after first 2 minutes
and then after every minute. Let
cool slightly. Serve warm.

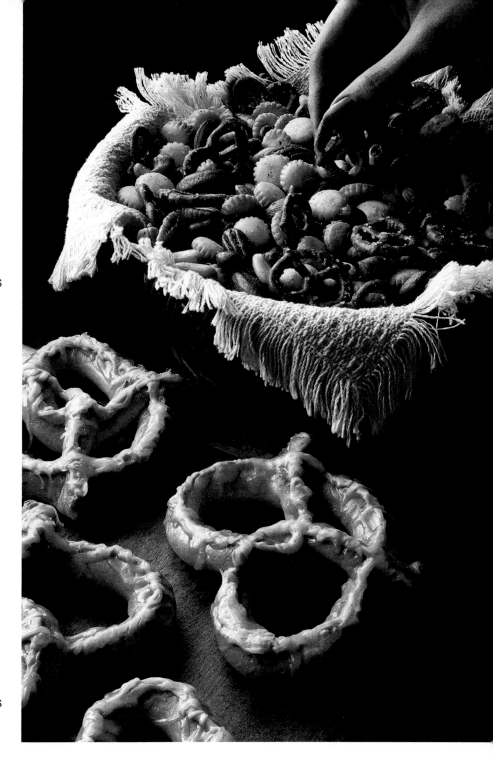

Hot Soft Pretzels ▲

4 soft pretzels
  Prepared mustard

¼ cup finely shredded Cheddar
   cheese

4 servings

Place pretzels on wax-paper-lined plate. Squeeze or spoon mustard
evenly on tops of pretzels. Sprinkle cheese evenly on tops of pretzels.
Press lightly, if necessary, so cheese adheres to mustard. Microwave
at 70% (Medium High) for 1½ to 2¼ minutes, or until pretzels are warm
and cheese is melted, rotating plate once.

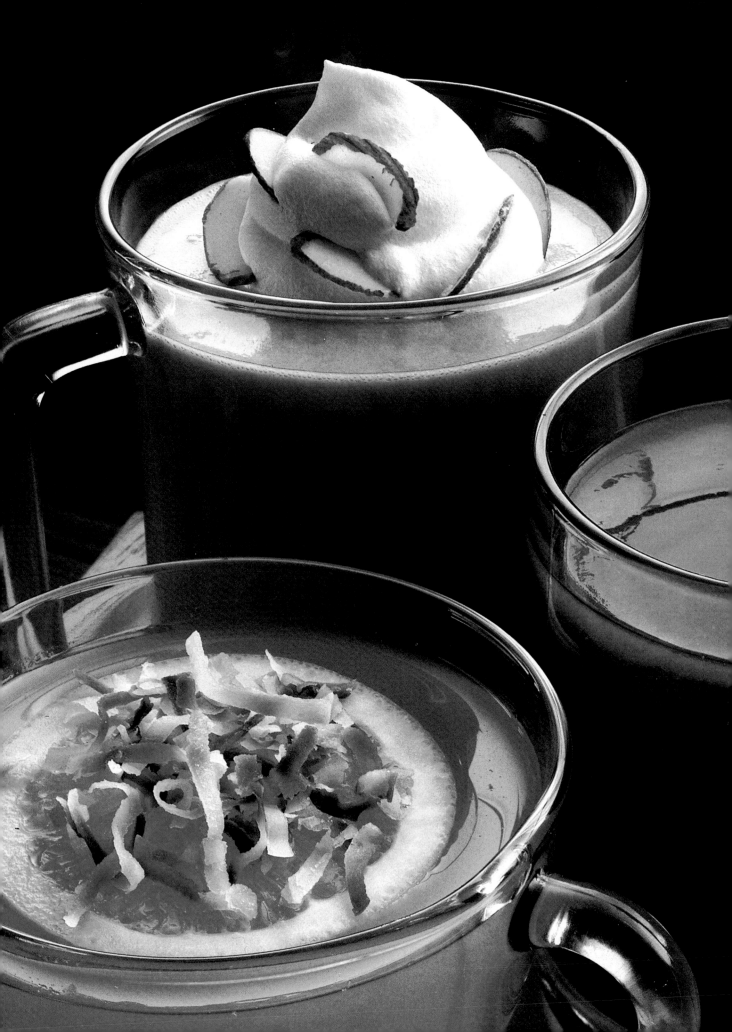

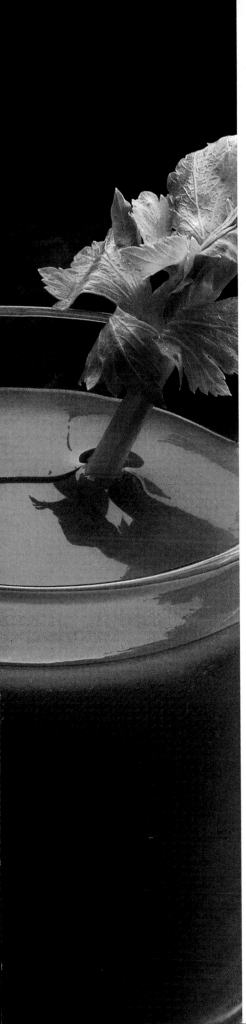

Beverages

◄ Mexican Hot Chocolate

⅔ cup sugar
½ cup cocoa
2 teaspoons ground cinnamon
½ cup hot water
4 cups milk
1 teaspoon vanilla
Prepared whipped topping
Sliced almonds

4 to 6 servings

In 3-quart casserole, combine sugar, cocoa and cinnamon. Add hot water. Mix well. Cover. Microwave at High for 2 to 3 minutes, or until mixture is hot, stirring once. Blend in milk.

Re-cover. Microwave at High for 8 to 11 minutes, or until mixture is hot but not boiling, stirring 2 or 3 times. Add vanilla. Serve hot, topped with whipped topping and almonds.

◄ Hot Pineapple Punch

1 can (46 oz.) pineapple juice
1 small orange, thinly sliced
¼ cup butter or margarine
1 to 2 tablespoons sugar
1 teaspoon rum extract
½ teaspoon ground cardamom
Toasted coconut (optional)

10 to 12 servings

In 8-cup measure, combine all ingredients, except coconut. Cover with plastic wrap. Microwave at High for 10 to 15 minutes, or until mixture is hot, stirring once or twice. Sprinkle each serving with toasted coconut before serving.

◄ Hot Bloody Mary

1¾ cups tomato juice
2 teaspoons lemon juice
¾ teaspoon Worcestershire sauce
¼ teaspoon celery salt
⅛ teaspoon red pepper sauce
2 tablespoons vodka
Fresh ground pepper
Celery stalks

2 servings

In 4-cup measure, combine tomato and lemon juices, Worcestershire sauce, celery salt and red pepper sauce. Cover with plastic wrap. Microwave at High for 3 to 4½ minutes, or until mixture is hot, stirring once. Stir in vodka. Divide evenly between 2 mugs. Top each drink with pepper and celery stalk.

Hearty Health Broth

1 can (10½ oz.) condensed beef broth
1 cup water
½ cup tomato juice
½ cup carrot juice
½ teaspoon onion powder
Dash dried thyme leaves
Dash pepper

4 servings

In 1½-quart casserole, combine all ingredients. Cover. Microwave at High for 7 to 10 minutes, or until mixture is hot, stirring twice. Serve in mugs. Garnish with celery stalk or whole green onion, if desired.

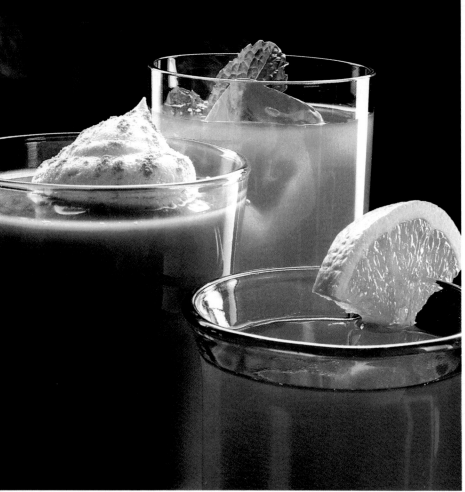

Cardamom-Spice Coffee ▲

1½ cups hot water
⅛ teaspoon ground allspice
⅛ teaspoon ground
    cardamom
 1 tablespoon instant coffee
    crystals
½ cup milk
 2 teaspoons sugar
    Prepared whipped topping

2 servings

Pour ¾ cup hot water into each
of 2 large coffee mugs. Sprinkle
evenly with allspice and cardamom. Microwave at High for 2½
to 4 minutes, or until water mixture
is hot. Stir 1½ teaspoons of coffee
crystals into each mug. Set aside.

In 1-cup measure, combine milk
and sugar. Microwave at High for
1¼ to 1¾ minutes, or until milk is
hot but not boiling, stirring once.
Pour milk mixture evenly into coffee mugs. Top with dollop of
whipped topping. Sprinkle with
additional cardamom, if desired.

Gingered Orange Tea ▲

 1 medium orange
 4 cups hot water
 1 tablespoon crystallized ginger
 4 tea bags

4 to 6 servings

Remove peel from orange. Set
orange aside. Using thin blade
of knife, cut away any white membrane from peel. Cut peel into thin
strips. Cut orange in half. Squeeze
halves and reserve juice.

In 2-quart measure, combine
orange peel strips and juice.
Add water and ginger. Cover
with plastic wrap. Microwave at
High for 8 to 10 minutes, or until
mixture is hot, stirring once. Add
tea bags and let steep for 3 to 5
minutes. Remove and discard
tea bags. To serve, strain tea into
cups. Serve tea iced, if desired.

◄ Peachy Iced Tea

 6 cups hot water
 1 can (5½ oz.) apricot nectar
 2 tablespoons lemon juice
 1 to 2 tablespoons packed
    brown sugar
 1 teaspoon grated lemon peel
 4 tea bags
1½ cups sliced frozen peaches

8 servings

In 2-quart measure, combine
water, apricot nectar, lemon juice,
brown sugar and lemon peel.
Cover with plastic wrap. Microwave at High for 11 to 14 minutes,
or until mixture is hot but not boiling, stirring once. Add tea bags.
Set aside.

Place peaches in 1-quart casserole. Cover. Microwave at 50%
(Medium) for 3½ to 5 minutes or
until peaches are defrosted, stirring once. Let stand for 3 to 5
minutes to complete defrosting.
In food processor or blender,
process peaches until smooth.

Remove and discard tea bags.
Stir peach mixture into tea. Chill
at least 2 hours. Serve over ice.
Garnish tea with lemon slice,
if desired.

Lemon & Spice Tea

 4 cups hot water
 2 teaspoons lemon juice
 1 teaspoon grated lemon peel
 6 whole cloves
 6 whole allspice
 4 tea bags
    Honey

4 servings

In 2-quart measure, combine
water, lemon juice, lemon peel,
cloves and allspice. Cover with
plastic wrap. Microwave at High
for 8 to 10 minutes, or until hot,
stirring twice. Add tea bags. Let
steep for 3 to 5 minutes. Remove
and discard tea bags. To serve,
strain tea into cups. Add honey
to taste.

Strawberry Margaritas ▼

2 cups frozen unsweetened
   strawberries
1½ cups water
½ cup sugar
1 can (6 oz.) frozen limeade
   concentrate
¾ cup tequila
¼ cup triple sec (orange
   liqueur)

4 to 6 servings

Place strawberries in 1-quart
casserole. Cover. Microwave at
50% (Medium) for 3½ to 5½ minutes, or until defrosted, stirring
once. Place in food processor or
blender. Process until smooth.
Set aside.

In 2-quart measure, combine
water and sugar. Microwave at
High for 2 to 3½ minutes, or until
water is hot and sugar is dissolved, stirring once. Set aside.

Remove lid from limeade can.
Place can in microwave oven.
Microwave at High for 30 to 45
seconds, or until limeade is defrosted. Pour into sugar mixture.
Add strawberries, tequila and
triple sec. Mix well.

Freeze margarita mixture for at
least 6 hours, or until slushy, stirring occasionally. Dip rim of
glass in water or lime juice, then
in sugar, before filling with frozen
margarita mixture.

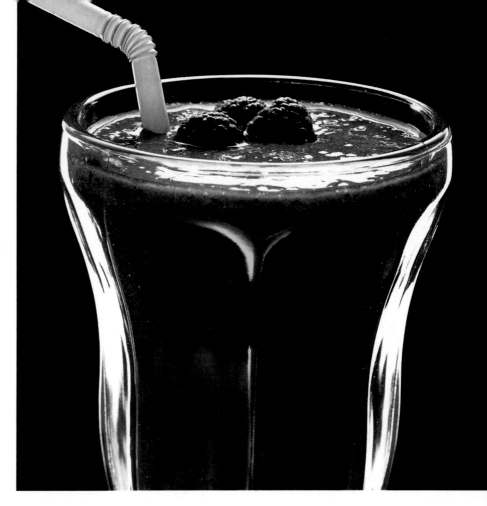

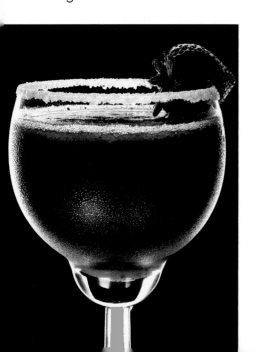

Refreshing Lime Cooler

1 can (12 oz.) frozen limeade
   concentrate
1 cup water
1 cup sugar
28 fresh or frozen strawberries
   Club soda or mineral water

28 cubes

Remove lid from limeade can.
Place can in microwave oven.
Microwave at High for 1 minute.
Set aside. In 1-quart measure,
combine water and sugar. Microwave at High for 2 to 3 minutes,
or until mixture is hot and sugar
is dissolved, stirring once or twice.
Add limeade and mix well.

Divide mixture evenly between
2 ice cube trays. Place 1 strawberry in each cube compartment.
Freeze for 5 to 6 hours, or until
cubes are firm. Loosen edges
of cubes with spatula. To serve,
place 2 or 3 cubes in each glass.
Pour club soda over cubes, and
mix slightly.

Tangy Raspberry Shake ▲

1 cup frozen unsweetened
   raspberries
¾ cup buttermilk
½ cup milk
1 tablespoon honey
2 tablespoons sweetened
   lemonade-flavored drink mix

2 servings

Place raspberries in 1-quart
casserole. Cover. Microwave at
50% (Medium) for 2 to 3 minutes,
or until defrosted, stirring once.
Place in blender or food processor. Add remaining ingredients.
Process until smooth and frothy.
Serve cold.

Tangy Blueberry Shake: Follow
recipe above, except substitute
1 cup frozen blueberries for
raspberries.

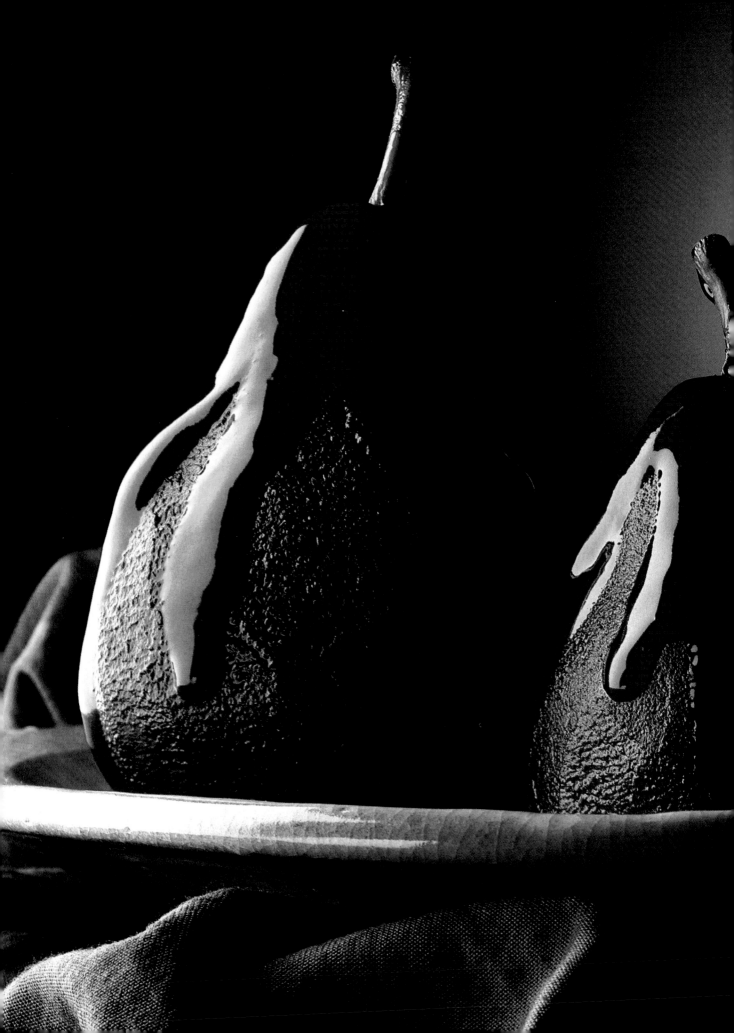

Fruits &
Sweet Snacks

Ruby Red Pears

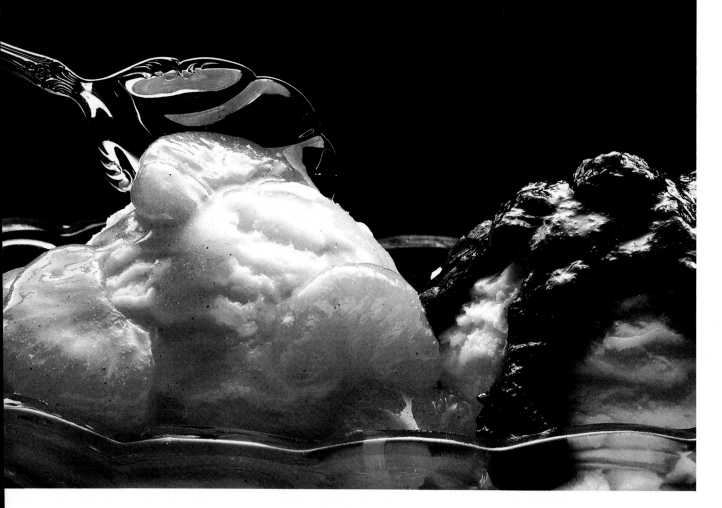

Mandarin Orange Sauce ▲

¼ cup packed brown sugar
2 teaspoons cornstarch
¼ teaspoon ground cinnamon
   Dash ground allspice
1 can (11 oz.) mandarin oranges,
   drained (reserve syrup)
¼ cup orange juice
1 teaspoon lemon juice
1 tablespoon butter or
   margarine

1½ cups

In 1-quart casserole, mix brown sugar, cornstarch, cinnamon and allspice. Blend in reserved mandarin orange syrup and the orange and lemon juices. Add butter. Microwave at High for 3½ to 5 minutes, or until mixture is thickened and translucent, stirring twice. Stir in orange segments. Serve warm over ice cream, pound cake, angel food cake, waffles or pancakes.

Ginger-spiced Applesauce

5 cups cored, peeled and thinly
   sliced apples
¼ cup water
2 tablespoons maple syrup
1 teaspoon grated fresh
   gingerroot
½ teaspoon grated orange peel
¼ teaspoon ground cinnamon
⅛ teaspoon ground nutmeg

4 to 6 servings

In 1½-quart casserole, combine all ingredients. Cover. Microwave at High for 9 to 15 minutes, or until apples are very soft, stirring once or twice. Let stand for 5 minutes. Place in food processor or blender. Process until smooth. Serve warm or chilled.

Rhubarb & Raspberry ▲ Dessert Sauce

3 cups frozen cut rhubarb
½ cup packed brown sugar
3 tablespoons water
¼ teaspoon ground allspice
1 cup frozen unsweetened
   raspberries
3 to 4 drops red food coloring

2 cups

In 2-quart casserole, combine rhubarb, brown sugar, water and allspice. Cover. Microwave at High for 13 to 18 minutes, or until rhubarb is very tender, stirring 2 or 3 times. Stir in raspberries and food coloring. Serve warm or chilled over ice cream, pound cake or angel food cake.

Pudding & Yogurt Cones ▶

1 pkg. (3.5 oz.) chocolate
    pudding and pie filling mix
2 cups milk
6 ice cream cones
1 container (8 oz.) strawberry
    yogurt
    Chopped pecans

6 servings

In 4-cup measure, combine
pudding mix and milk. Mix well.
Microwave at High for 6 to 9 minutes, or until mixture thickens
and bubbles, stirring every 2
minutes. Place plastic wrap
directly on surface of pudding.
Chill completely.

Fill each cone one-third full with
pudding. Layer yogurt evenly over
pudding. Fill cones with remaining pudding, mounding slightly
at tops. Sprinkle tops with pecans. Serve immediately.

Banana Macaroon Gratin

1 pkg. (3⅛ oz.) coconut cream
    pudding and pie filling mix
2 cups milk
3 medium bananas, sliced

Topping:
1 cup crumbled macaroon
    cookies (about 6)
½ cup chocolate chips
¼ cup flaked coconut

4 to 6 servings

In 4-cup measure, combine
pudding mix and milk. Mix well.
Microwave at High for 6 to 9 minutes, or until mixture thickens and
bubbles, stirring every 2 minutes.
Add banana slices. Pour mixture
into 1-quart gratin dish or shallow
1-quart casserole.

In small mixing bowl, combine
topping ingredients. Sprinkle
evenly over pudding mixture.
Microwave at High for 3 to 4 minutes, or until chocolate is glossy,
rotating dish once. Let cool slightly
before serving.

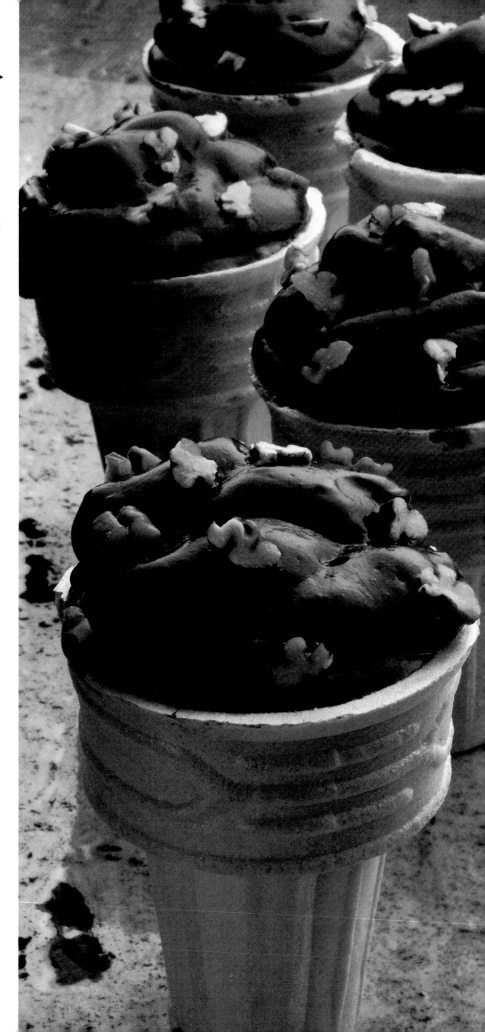

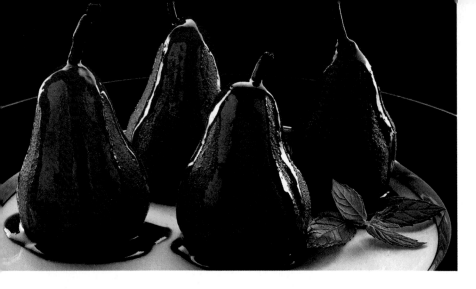

Ruby Red Pears

    1 cup red port wine
 1/3 cup sugar
    2 slices orange
    1 stick cinnamon
    4 whole cloves
 1/2 teaspoon red food coloring
    4 pears (about 8 oz. each)
    2 teaspoons cornstarch
      Sweetened whipped cream
      (optional)

4 servings

How to Microwave Ruby Red Pears

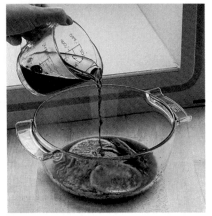

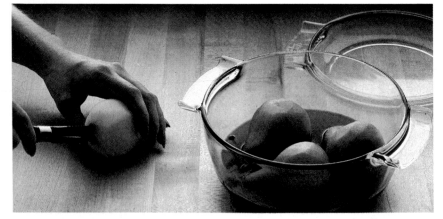

Combine wine, sugar, orange slices, cinnamon and cloves in 2-quart casserole. Cover. Microwave at High for 3 to 4 minutes, or until sugar dissolves, stirring once or twice. Add food coloring. Mix well. Set aside.

Peel pears. Core from bottom, being careful not to cut through stem end. Roll pears in wine mixture to coat. Cover. Microwave at High for 13 to 20 minutes, or until tender, turning pears over and basting with wine mixture 2 or 3 times.

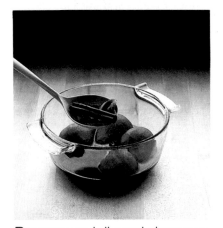

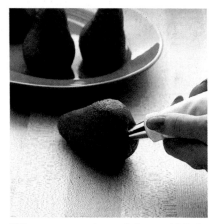

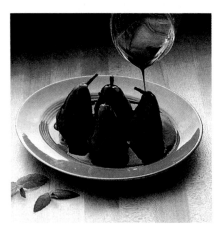

Remove and discard cinnamon stick, cloves and orange slices. Re-cover pears. Chill in wine mixture for about 4 hours. Drain wine mixture, reserving 1 cup. Blend cornstarch into reserved mixture.

Microwave wine mixture at High for 3½ to 4½ minutes, or until mixture is thickened and translucent, stirring once or twice. Pipe whipped cream into pear centers.

Arrange pears on serving platter. Pour glaze evenly over pears. Garnish with sweetened whipped cream and mint leaves, if desired.

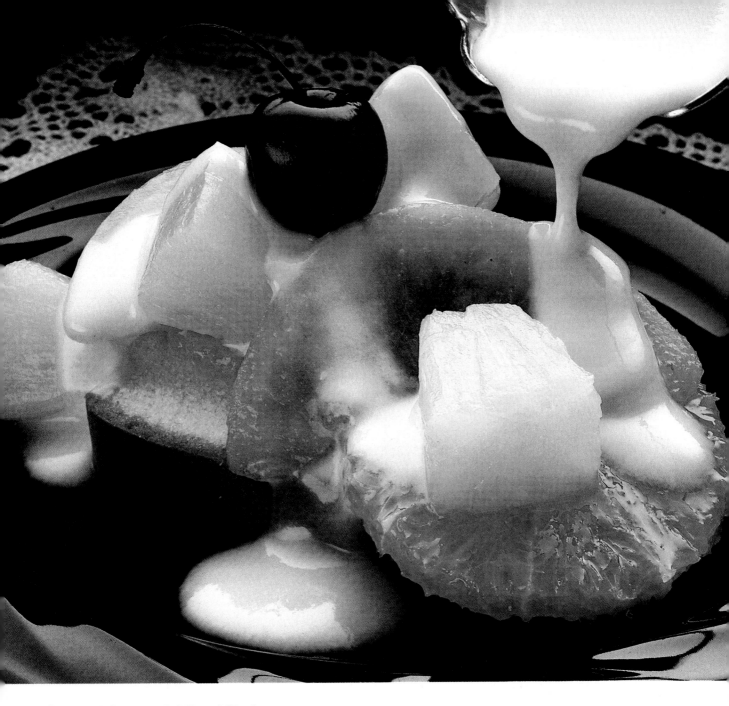

Custard Sauce & Mixed Fruit

¼ cup sugar
2 teaspoons all-purpose flour
½ teaspoon grated lemon peel
1 cup milk
2 eggs, beaten
1 medium orange
4 thin slices angel food cake or
   pound cake
1 can (8 oz.) pineapple chunks,
   drained
1 medium peach, peeled and
   sliced
4 maraschino cherries

4 servings

In 2-cup measure, combine sugar, flour and lemon peel. Mix well. Blend in milk. Microwave at High for 3½ to 5½ minutes, or until mixture boils, stirring 2 or 3 times. Stir small amount of hot mixture gradually into eggs. Blend eggs back into hot mixture. Microwave at 50% (Medium) for 30 seconds to 1 minute, or until mixture thickens slightly, stirring once. Place plastic wrap directly on surface of custard sauce. Chill completely.

Using sharp knife, peel skin and white membrane from orange. Cut orange crosswise into 8 slices. Place 1 cake slice on each of 4 dessert plates. Top each with 2 orange slices, then layer evenly with pineapple and peach slices. Pour custard sauce evenly over desserts. Garnish each serving with maraschino cherry.

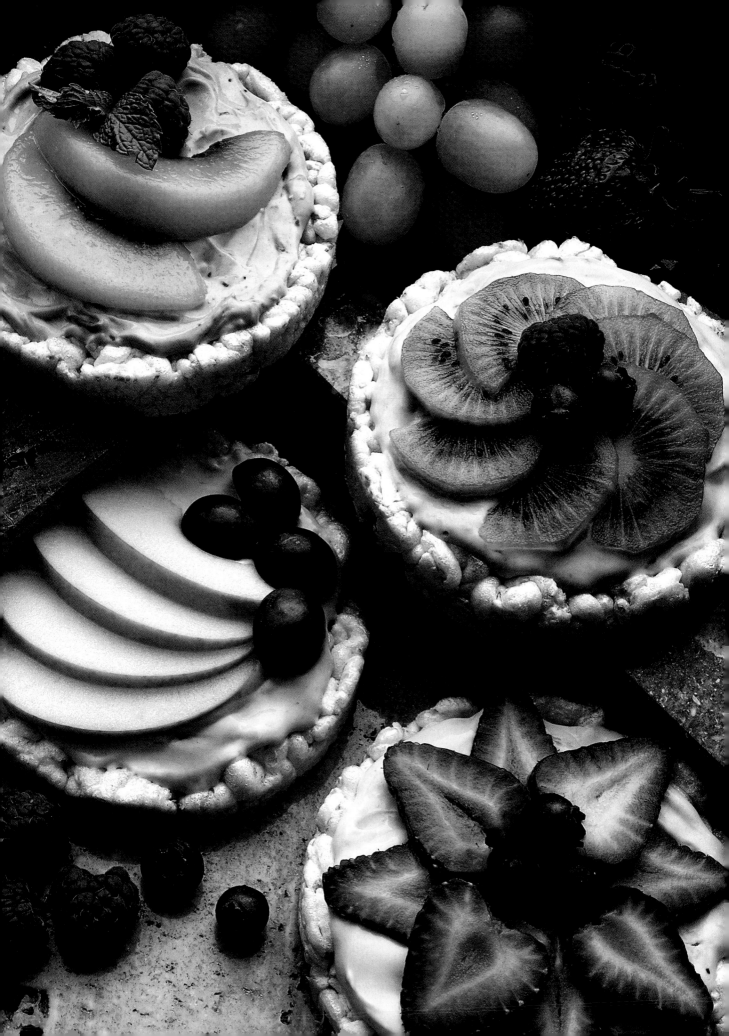

◄ Crispy Fruit & Cheese Rounds

4 oz. cream cheese
1 tablespoon strawberry, raspberry or blueberry jam
4 rice cakes

Toppings:
  Sliced fresh strawberries, peaches, apples, bananas, pears or kiwifruit
  Raspberries, blueberries or grapes

4 servings

Place cream cheese in small mixing bowl. Microwave at High for 45 seconds to 1 minute, or until softened. Add jam. Mix well. Spread one-fourth of cheese mixture on each rice cake. Top with desired fruit.

Mini Savarins

¼ cup sugar
¼ cup water
1 teaspoon butter or margarine
½ teaspoon lemon juice
1 tablespoon rum
4 individual sponge cake cups
¼ cup seedless green grapes
¼ cup seedless red grapes
1 orange slice, cut into quarters
¼ cup orange marmalade

4 servings

In 1-cup measure, combine sugar, water, butter and lemon juice. Microwave at High for 1½ to 2 minutes, or until mixture boils, stirring once. Microwave at High for 1 minute longer. Stir in rum. Set aside.

Place 1 cake in each of 4 dessert dishes. Pierce cakes with wooden skewer. Slowly pour rum syrup evenly over each cake. Top cakes evenly with fruit. Set aside.

In small dish, microwave marmalade at 50% (Medium) for 1½ to 2 minutes, or until melted, stirring once. Brush evenly over savarins. Chill for at least 1 hour.

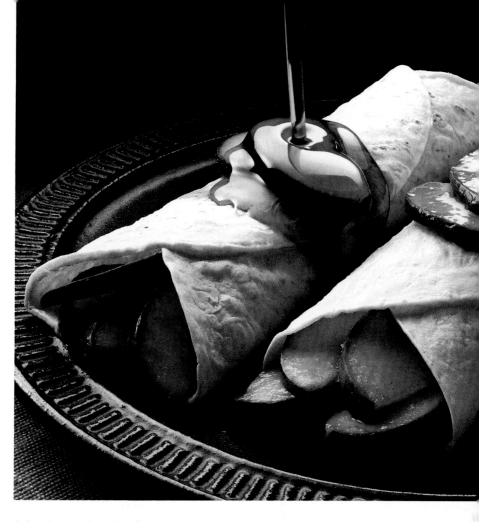

Mexican Apple Strudel ▲

2½ cups sliced apples
¼ cup packed brown sugar
1 tablespoon all-purpose flour
¼ teaspoon apple pie spice
  Dash salt
1 teaspoon lemon juice
1 tablespoon butter or margarine
2 flour tortillas (8-inch)
¼ cup maple syrup (optional)

2 servings

In 1-quart casserole, combine apples, brown sugar, flour, apple pie spice and salt. Toss to coat. Drizzle with lemon juice. Add butter. Cover. Microwave at High for 3½ to 5½ minutes, or until apples are tender and sauce is thickened, stirring once.

Spoon apple mixture evenly down centers of tortillas. Roll up tortillas, enclosing filling. In 1-cup measure, microwave maple syrup at High for 15 to 30 seconds, or until warm. Pour over tortillas.

Fresh Fruit Compote

2 cups fresh strawberries, hulled
1 cup fresh blueberries
1 kiwifruit, peeled and thinly sliced
2 tablespoons packed brown sugar
1 tablespoon cornstarch
½ teaspoon grated orange or lime peel
¼ teaspoon ground cinnamon
1¼ cups orange juice

4 servings

Arrange fruit evenly in each of 4 dessert dishes. Set aside. In small mixing bowl, combine brown sugar, cornstarch, orange peel and cinnamon. Blend in orange juice. Microwave at High for 3 to 6 minutes, or until mixture is thickened and translucent, stirring 2 or 3 times. Pour sauce evenly over fruit. Chill for 2 to 3 hours.

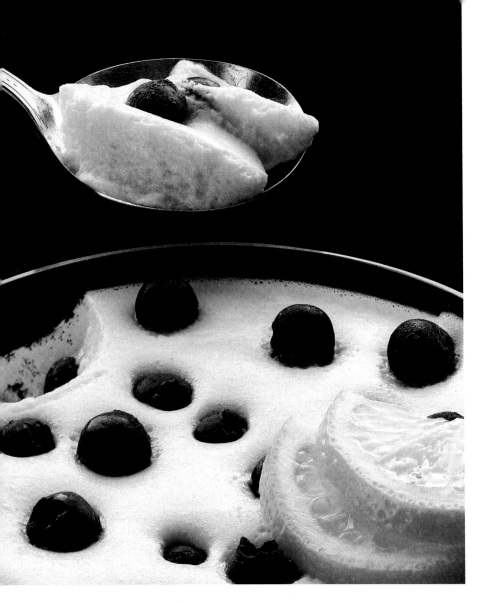

Lemon Blueberry Mousse

 2 eggs, separated
 ¾ cup evaporated skimmed
    milk
 ½ cup water
 ¼ cup lemon juice
 ¼ cup sugar
 1 envelope (.25 oz.)
    unflavored gelatin
 1 teaspoon grated lemon peel
 ½ cup prepared whipped
    topping
 1½ cups fresh blueberries,
    divided

6 to 8 servings

How to Microwave Lemon Blueberry Mousse

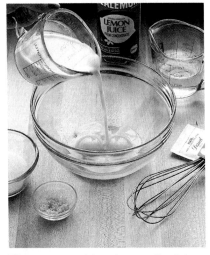

Place egg whites in small mixing bowl. Set aside. Place egg yolks in medium mixing bowl. Add milk, water, lemon juice, sugar, gelatin and lemon peel. Blend well.

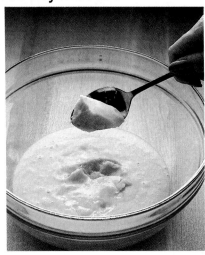

Microwave at 50% (Medium) for 8 to 14 minutes, or just until mixture boils, stirring 3 times with a whisk. Chill until mixture is consistency of pudding, about 1½ hours, stirring occasionally.

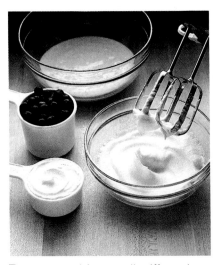

Beat egg whites until stiff peaks form. Fold into milk mixture. Fold in whipped topping and 1 cup blueberries. Sprinkle with remaining ½ cup blueberries. Chill until set, about 1 hour. Garnish with lemon slices, if desired.

46

Raspberry Bavarian

1 cup hot water
1 pkg. (0.3 oz.) low-calorie
　 raspberry-flavored gelatin
¾ cup cold water
2 cups frozen unsweetened
　 raspberries
1 egg white
1½ cups prepared whipped
　 topping, divided

6 servings

Place hot water in 2-cup measure. Microwave at High for 2 to 2¾ minutes, or until water boils. Place gelatin in medium mixing bowl. Stir in boiling water. Stir to dissolve gelatin. Mix in cold water. Chill until gelatin is soft-set, about 1 hour.

Place raspberries in 1-quart casserole. Cover. Microwave at 50% (Medium) for 3 to 5 minutes, or until raspberries are defrosted, stirring once. Reserve 6 whole berries for garnishing, if desired. Stir raspberries into gelatin. Set aside.

Place egg white in small mixing bowl. Beat at high speed of an electric mixer until stiff peaks form. Fold into gelatin mixture. Fold 1 cup whipped topping into gelatin mixture. Spoon into each of 6 stemmed glasses or dessert dishes. Top evenly with remaining ½ cup whipped topping. Garnish with raspberries. Serve immediately, or chill for 1 hour for firmer texture.

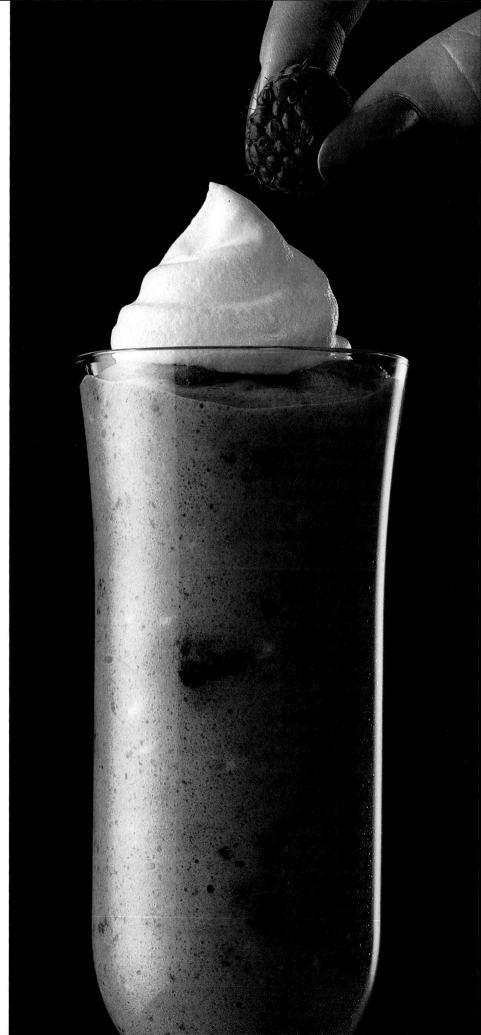

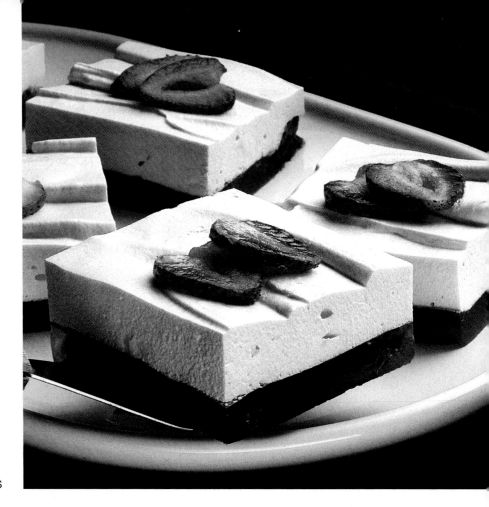

Fluffy Strawberry Layers

　　Vegetable cooking spray
¾　cup water
2　envelopes (.25 oz. each)
　　　unflavored gelatin
1　pkg. (10 oz.) frozen
　　　strawberry halves in syrup
½　cup orange juice
¼　cup sugar
4　to 5 drops red food coloring
2　cups prepared whipped
　　　topping

9 servings

How to Microwave Fluffy Strawberry Layers

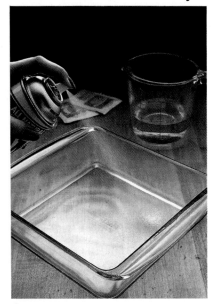

Spray 9-inch square baking dish with vegetable cooking spray. Set aside. In 2-cup measure, microwave water at High for 2 to 2¾ minutes, or until boiling. Add gelatin. Stir thoroughly to dissolve. Set aside.

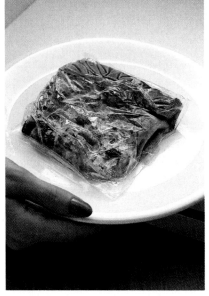

Place frozen strawberries on plate. Microwave at High for 1¾ to 2¾ minutes, or until completely defrosted. Empty pouch into medium mixing bowl. Stir in orange juice, sugar and food coloring. Mix well to dissolve sugar. Stir in gelatin mixture.

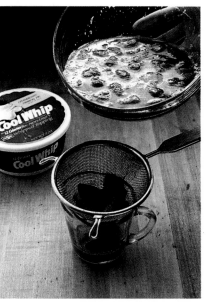

Drain and reserve ½ cup liquid from strawberries. Place reserved liquid in small mixing bowl. Set aside. Pour strawberries and remaining liquid into prepared dish. Blend whipped topping into reserved liquid. Spread evenly over strawberry mixture. Chill until firm, about 2 hours.

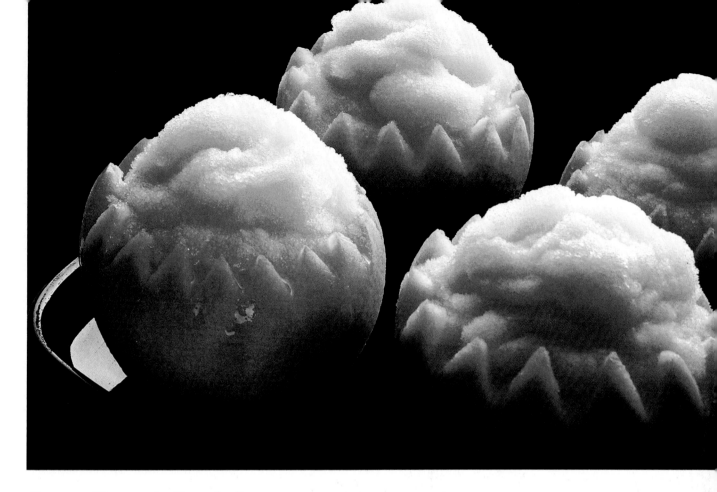

Orange-Pineapple Snowballs ▲

3 oranges, cut in half crosswise
1 can (6 oz.) pineapple juice
½ cup water
¼ cup sugar

6 servings

Using fruit knife, loosen orange pulp and remove from orange halves. Place pulp in wire strainer over medium mixing bowl. Set aside. Arrange orange shells cut-side-up on baking sheet. Place in freezer. Mash orange pulp and strain to yield 1 cup orange juice. Add pineapple juice. Set aside. In 1-cup measure, combine water and sugar. Microwave at High for 1½ to 2 minutes, or until sugar dissolves, stirring once. Add water and sugar mixture to juice mixture. Mix well. Freeze mixture overnight, or until firm. Break apart and place in food processor. Process until smooth. Spoon icy mixture evenly into frozen orange shells. Freeze.

Gingersnap-Apricot Freeze

¼ cup butter or margarine
1 cup finely crushed
   gingersnaps
1 can (5½ oz.) apricot nectar
½ cup nonfat dry milk powder
2 egg whites
¼ cup sugar
1 can (16 oz.) apricot halves,
   chopped

9 servings

Place butter in 9-inch square baking dish. Microwave at High for 1¼ to 1½ minutes, or until butter melts. Add cookie crumbs. Mix well. Reserve 2 tablespoons crumb mixture for topping. Press remaining crumb mixture into an even layer in bottom of dish. Microwave at High for 1½ minutes, rotating dish once. Cool completely.

In large mixing bowl, combine apricot nectar, milk powder and egg whites. Beat at high speed of an electric mixer until mixture becomes light and foamy, about 3 minutes. Gradually beat in sugar. Fold in chopped apricots. Pour mixture over prepared crust. Sprinkle with reserved crumbs. Freeze until mixture is firm, 4 to 6 hours. Remove from freezer 10 minutes before serving.

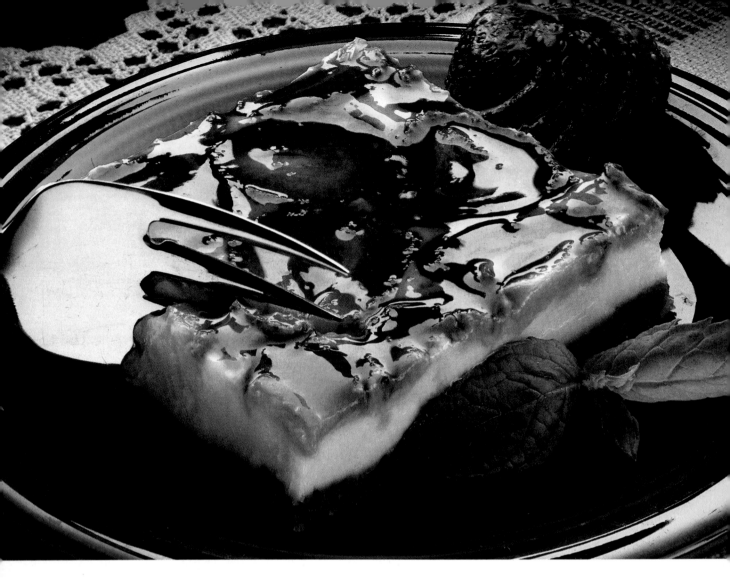

Strawberry-Cheese Dessert ▲

⅓ cup butter or margarine
¾ cup graham cracker crumbs
2 tablespoons sugar

Filling:
1 pkg. (8 oz.) cream cheese

¼ cup sour cream
1 egg
3 tablespoons sugar
1 tablespoon all-purpose flour
1 cup sliced fresh strawberries
⅓ cup strawberry jelly

9 servings

Place butter in 9-inch square baking dish. Microwave at High for 1½ to 1¾ minutes, or until butter melts. Add graham cracker crumbs and sugar. Mix well. Press into an even layer in bottom of dish. Microwave at High for 1½ minutes, rotating dish once. Set aside.

In medium mixing bowl, microwave cream cheese at 50% (Medium) for 1½ to 3 minutes, or until softened. Add sour cream, egg, sugar and flour. Beat at medium speed of an electric mixer until mixture is smooth.

Pour cream cheese mixture over crust. Top evenly with strawberries. Microwave at 50% (Medium) for 8 to 12 minutes, or until center is set, rotating dish 2 or 3 times. Chill until completely set, about 1 hour.

Place jelly in small mixing bowl. Microwave at High for 1½ to 2 minutes, or until jelly melts, stirring once. Spoon evenly over dessert. Before serving, chill for 30 minutes.

Yogurt & Fruit Candy Bars

1 lb. white candy coating, broken into squares
⅓ cup plain low-fat yogurt
1 pkg. (6 oz.) diced mixed dried fruit
2 cups crisp rice cereal
½ cup slivered almonds

36 bars

Butter a 9-inch square baking dish. Set aside. Place candy coating in 2-quart casserole. Microwave at 50% (Medium) for 4 to 8 minutes, or until candy coating is melted and can be stirred smooth, stirring twice. Blend in yogurt. Mix in remaining ingredients. Spread evenly into prepared baking dish. Chill until firm, at least 1 hour. Cut into 36 bars. Store in refrigerator.

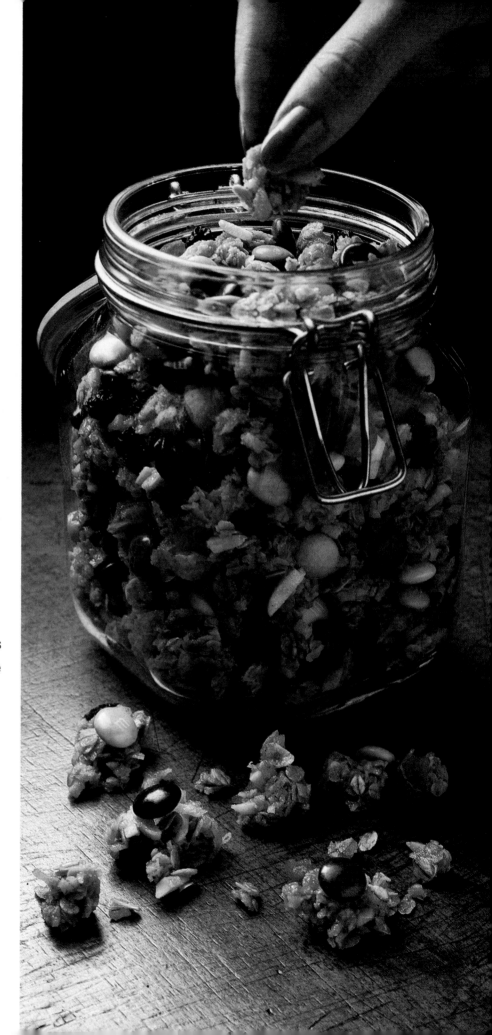

Crunchy Granola

1½ cups old-fashioned rolled
    oats
⅓ cup flaked coconut
¼ cup slivered almonds
⅓ cup honey
3 tablespoons packed brown
    sugar
2 tablespoons butter or
    margarine
2 tablespoons dark corn
    syrup
1 teaspoon vanilla
¼ cup dried apricot halves,
    chopped
¼ cup raisins
½ cup candy-coated plain
    chocolate pieces

4 cups

In medium mixing bowl, combine oats, coconut and almonds. Mix well. Set aside. In 4-cup measure, combine honey, brown sugar, butter and corn syrup. Microwave at High for 2 to 4 minutes, or until mixture boils, stirring once. Stir in vanilla.

Pour hot mixture over oat mixture. Toss to coat. Microwave at High for 5½ to 8 minutes, or until mixture appears dry and begins to stiffen, stirring 2 or 3 times. Add apricots and raisins. Spread granola in an even layer on wax-paper-lined baking sheet. Cool. Sprinkle with chocolate pieces. Break into small pieces. Store in airtight container.

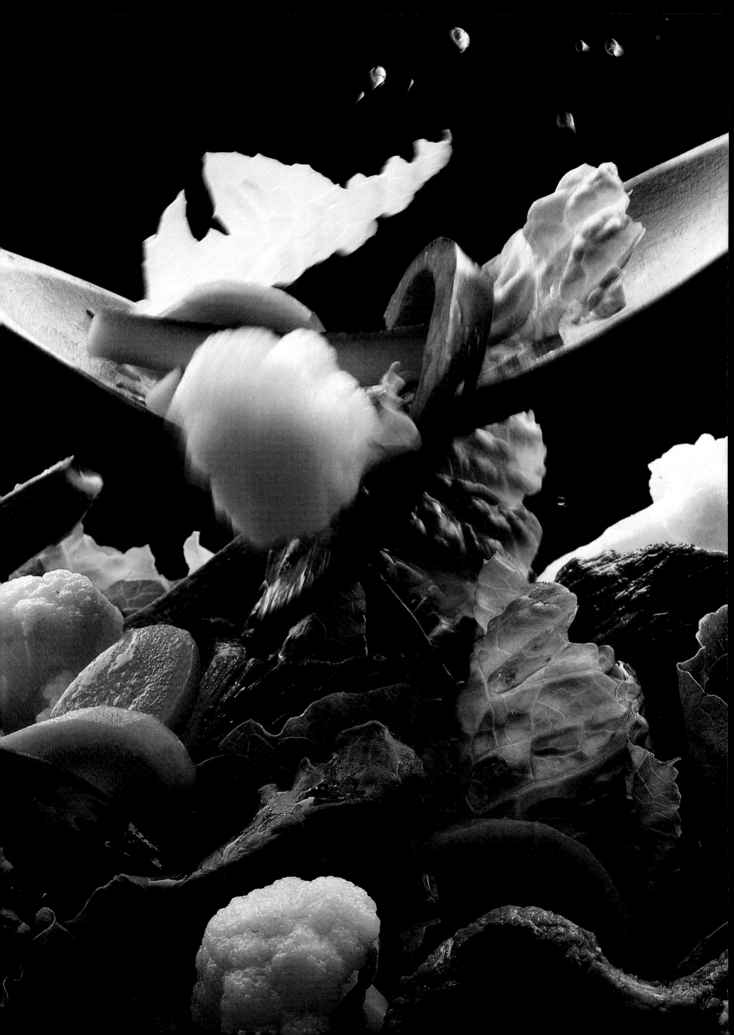

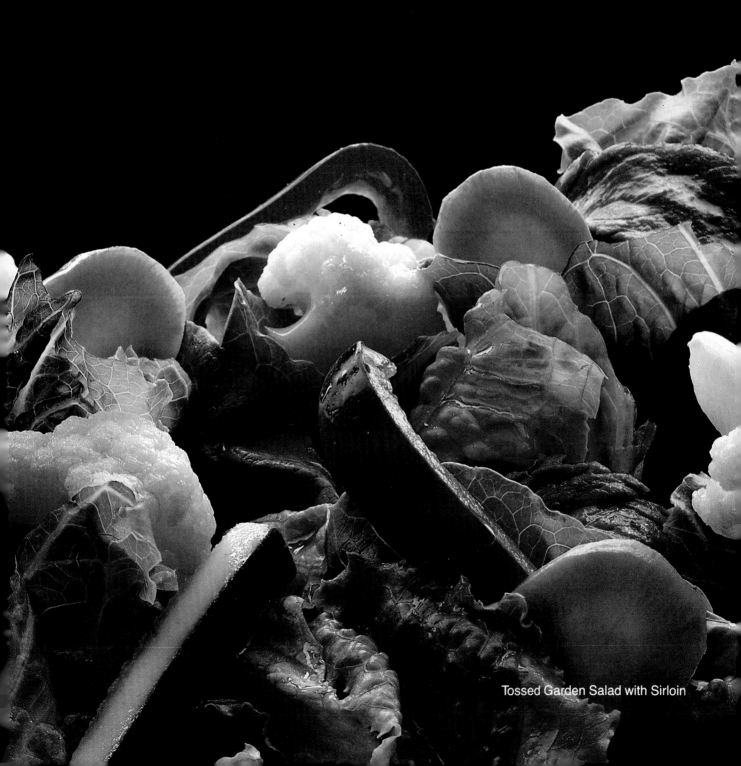

Salads, Soups & Sandwiches

Tossed Garden Salad with Sirloin

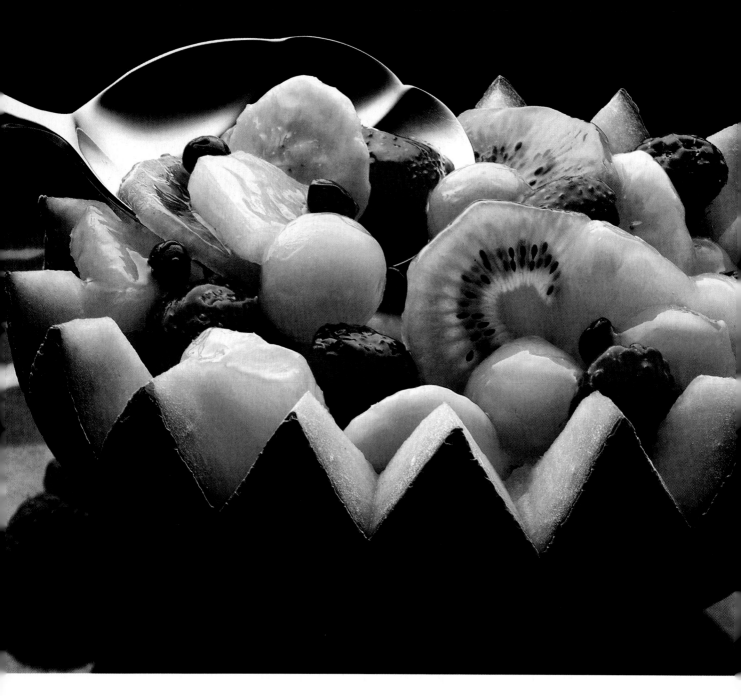

Apple-Ginger Fruit Salad

3 tablespoons sugar
2 teaspoons cornstarch
  Dash salt
½ cup apple juice
½ teaspoon lemon juice
¼ teaspoon grated fresh
  gingerroot
1 medium cantaloupe or
  honeydew melon (about
  3¾ lbs.)*
8 to 10 cups cut-up mixed fruit
  (fresh, canned or frozen)

10 to 12 servings

In 2-cup measure, mix sugar, cornstarch and salt. Blend in apple juice. Stir in lemon juice and gingerroot. Microwave at High for 2½ to 3½ minutes, or until mixture is thickened and translucent, stirring once or twice. Cool.

Cut melon in half. Cut edge of each half with decorative zigzagged or scalloped pattern, if desired. Using small spoon or melon baller, scoop out centers of melon halves to form shells. Reserve melon balls to include in salad, as desired. Set shells aside. Combine fruit in large mixing bowl. Add dressing, stirring gently to coat. Spoon fruit salad into melon shells to serve. Refill with additional fruit salad as needed.

*For variety, use one cantaloupe half and one honeydew melon half for salad shells. Reserve remaining melon halves for future use.

Confetti Rice Salad

- 2 cups hot water
- 1 cup uncooked long-grain white rice
- 2 teaspoons dried parsley flakes
- 1 teaspoon instant chicken bouillon granules
- 2 tablespoons butter or margarine
- ½ cup whole blanched almonds
- 2 cups fresh broccoli flowerets
- 2 tablespoons water
- 1 cup frozen corn
- ¼ cup raisins
- ½ cup julienne red pepper (1½ × ¼-inch strips)

Dressing:
- 3 tablespoons vinegar
- 3 tablespoons sugar
- 3 tablespoons vegetable oil
- ½ teaspoon salt
- ½ teaspoon dry mustard

6 to 8 servings

In 2-quart casserole, combine hot water, rice, parsley and chicken bouillon granules. Cover. Microwave at High for 5 minutes. Microwave at 50% (Medium) for 12 to 15 minutes longer, or until rice is tender and liquid is absorbed. Let stand, covered, for 5 minutes.

In medium mixing bowl, microwave butter at High for 45 seconds to 1 minute, or until melted. Add almonds. Toss to coat. Microwave at High for 3 to 4 minutes, or just until almonds begin to brown, stirring once. Remove almonds from butter. Drain on paper towels. Set aside.

In 1-quart casserole, place broccoli and 2 tablespoons water. Cover. Microwave at High for 2 to 3 minutes, or until broccoli is very hot and color brightens, stirring once. Rinse with cold water. Drain. Add almonds, broccoli, corn, raisins and red pepper strips to rice mixture. In 2-cup measure, blend all dressing ingredients. Mix well. Pour over salad. Toss to coat. Cover and chill for 2 to 3 hours before serving.

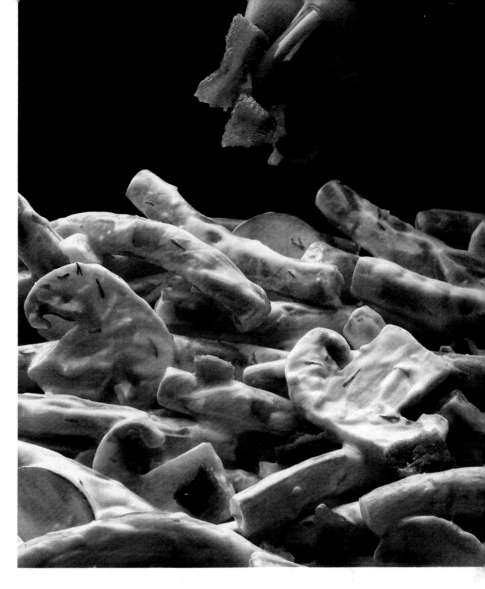

Fresh Green Bean Salad ▲

- 1 lb. fresh green beans
- ½ cup water
- ½ cup sliced fresh mushrooms
- ⅓ cup thinly sliced radishes
- 1 tablespoon sliced green onion
- 4 slices bacon

Dressing:
- ⅓ cup sour cream
- ¼ cup mayonnaise
- 1 tablespoon milk
- 1 teaspoon prepared horseradish
- ¼ teaspoon salt
- ¼ teaspoon sugar
- ¼ teaspoon dried dill weed

4 servings

Trim ends of green beans. Place beans in 1½-quart casserole. Add water. Cover. Microwave at High for 10 to 15 minutes, or until beans are tender-crisp, stirring once or twice. Rinse with cold water. Drain. Place in medium mixing bowl. Add mushrooms, radishes and onion. Cover. Chill for at least 1 hour.

Arrange bacon slices on roasting rack. Cover with paper towel. Microwave at High for 3 to 6 minutes, or until brown and crisp, rotating rack once. Cool slightly and crumble. Set aside. In small bowl, combine all dressing ingredients. Mix well. Pour over green bean salad. Toss to coat. Sprinkle top with crumbled bacon.

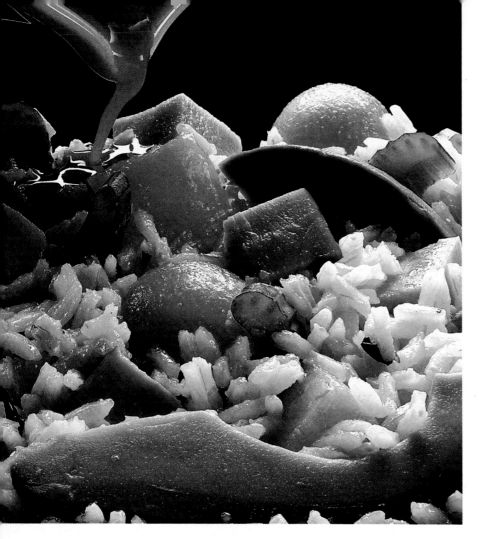

Festive Turkey Rice Salad ▲

2   cups hot water
1   cup uncooked long-grain
      white rice
1   teaspoon dried parsley flakes
1   teaspoon grated orange peel
1   teaspoon grated lemon peel
1   teaspoon instant chicken
      bouillon granules
½   teaspoon salt
1   cup cubed cooked turkey
      (½-inch cubes)
1   cup small cantaloupe chunks
      or balls

1   can (8 oz.) pineapple chunks,
      drained
½   cup sliced celery
1   avocado, peeled and sliced

Dressing:
¼   cup vegetable oil
2   tablespoons orange juice
1   tablespoon vinegar
½   teaspoon sugar
¼   teaspoon dry mustard
¼   teaspoon paprika

6 to 8 servings

In 2-quart casserole, combine water, rice, parsley, grated orange and lemon peels, chicken bouillon granules and salt. Cover. Microwave at High for 5 minutes. Microwave at 50% (Medium) for 12 to 15 minutes longer, or until liquid is absorbed. Let stand, covered, for 5 minutes. Stir. Re-cover. Chill for at least 3 hours.

Place rice in large mixing bowl. Add turkey, cantaloupe, pineapple, celery and avocado. Set aside. In 1-cup measure, blend all dressing ingredients. Pour over salad and mix well. Serve immediately, or cover and chill before serving.

Chicken Taco Salad

2½ to 3-lb. broiler-fryer chicken,
      cut into quarters, skin
      removed
¾   teaspoon dried oregano
      leaves
½   teaspoon ground cumin
⅛   teaspoon ground cinnamon
1   can (16 oz.) pinto beans,
      drained
1   small onion, chopped
½   cup chopped green pepper
½   cup taco sauce
5   cups shredded lettuce
1   medium tomato, cut into
      wedges
      Black olives (optional)
      Sour cream or guacamole

6 to 8 servings

In 10-inch square casserole, arrange chicken with thickest portions toward outside. Set aside. In small bowl, combine oregano, cumin and cinnamon. Mix well and sprinkle evenly over chicken. Cover. Microwave at High for 13 to 19 minutes, or until chicken near bone is no longer pink and juices run clear, rearranging once. Cool slightly. Remove meat from bones and cut into bite-size pieces.

In medium mixing bowl, combine chicken, beans, onion and green pepper. Add taco sauce. Mix well. Spread shredded lettuce on serving platter. Mound chicken mixture on lettuce. Garnish with tomato wedges and black olives. Top chicken mixture with sour cream.

Chicken Platter with Orange-Basil Dressing

Dressing:

½ cup ricotta cheese
¼ cup mayonnaise
¼ cup snipped fresh basil
3 tablespoons olive oil
1 teaspoon grated orange peel
⅛ teaspoon salt
Dash dry mustard

2 boneless whole chicken
  breasts (10 to 12 oz. each),
  split in half, skin removed
1 tablespoon Dijon mustard
2 teaspoons water
1 head Bibb lettuce, torn into
  bite-size pieces
1 cup sliced fresh mushrooms
½ cup salted cashews
  Orange slices (optional)

4 to 6 servings

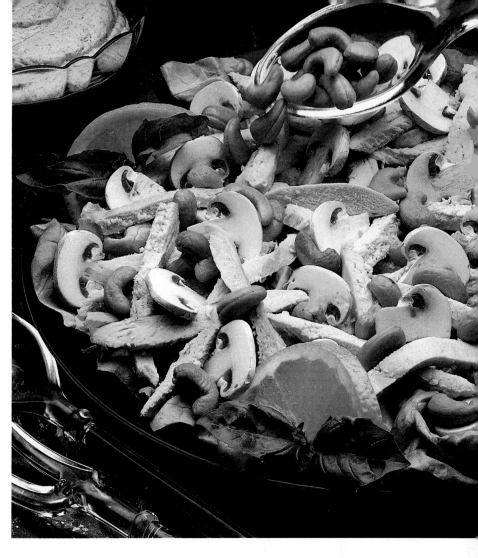

How to Microwave Chicken Platter with Orange-Basil Dressing

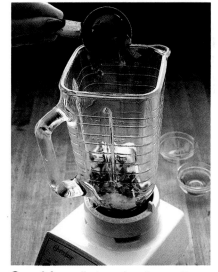

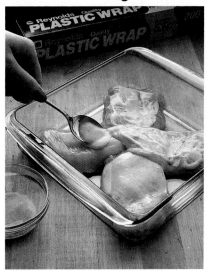

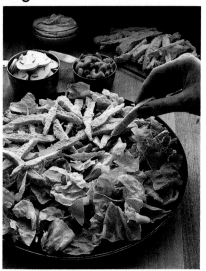

Combine all dressing ingredients in blender or food processor. Process until smooth. Place in bowl. Cover and chill. In 9-inch square baking dish, arrange chicken with thickest portions toward outside.

Blend mustard and water in small bowl. Spoon evenly over chicken. Cover with plastic wrap. Microwave at 70% (Medium High) for 9 to 12 minutes, or until chicken is no longer pink and juices run clear, rotating once.

Cut chicken into thin julienne strips. Line large serving platter with lettuce. Arrange chicken, mushrooms and cashews on lettuce. Garnish with orange slices. Serve with dressing.

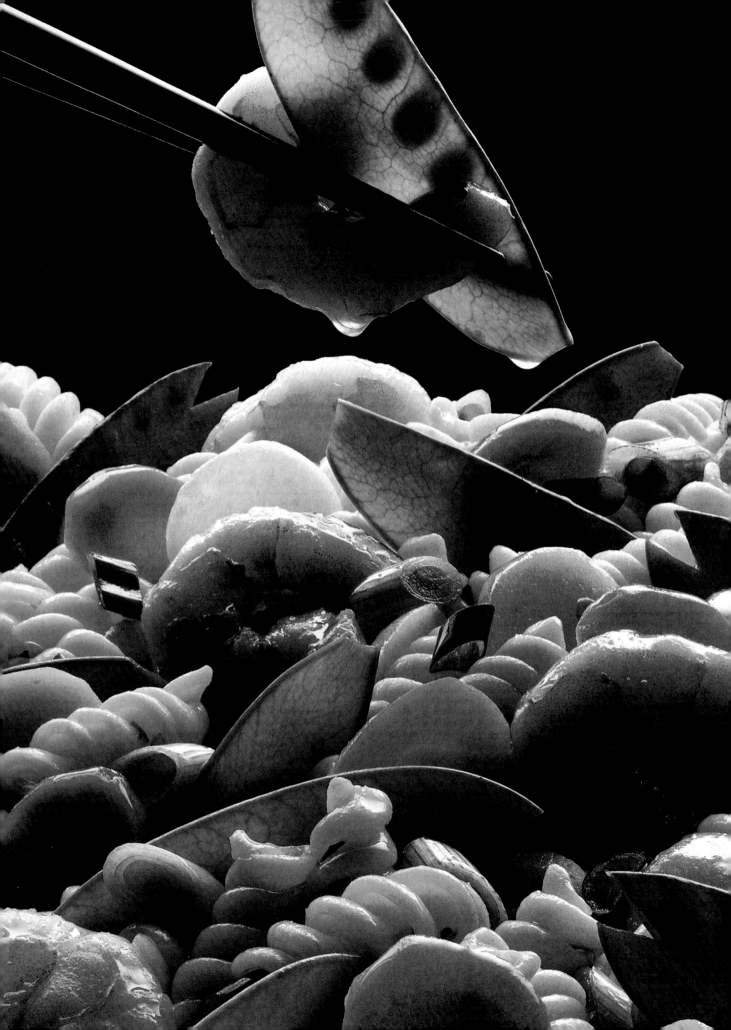

◄ Oriental Shrimp & Pasta Salad

½ lb. medium shrimp, shelled and deveined
8 oz. uncooked rotini pasta
1 cup diagonally sliced carrots (⅛-inch thick)
4 oz. fresh pea pods
2 tablespoons water
1 can (8 oz.) sliced water chestnuts, rinsed and drained
¼ cup sliced green onions

Dressing:
2 tablespoons vegetable oil
2 tablespoons soy sauce
2 tablespoons rice wine vinegar
2 teaspoons sesame seed
1 teaspoon sesame oil
1 teaspoon sugar
¼ teaspoon crushed red pepper flakes

4 servings

Place shrimp in 1½-quart casserole. Cover. Microwave at 70% (Medium High) for 2½ to 4 minutes, or until shrimp are firm, stirring once or twice. Rinse with cold water. Drain and set aside. Prepare pasta as directed on package. Rinse with cold water. Drain and set aside.

In 2-quart casserole, combine carrots, pea pods and water. Cover. Microwave at High for 3 to 4 minutes, or until vegetables are very hot and colors brighten, stirring once or twice. Rinse with cold water. Drain. In same 2-quart casserole, combine carrots, pea pods, cooked pasta, shrimp, water chestnuts and onions. Set aside.

In 2-cup measure, combine dressing ingredients. Microwave at High for 30 seconds to 1 minute, or until dressing is warm and sugar is dissolved, stirring once. Pour dressing over pasta mixture. Toss to coat. Cover and chill for 3 to 4 hours.

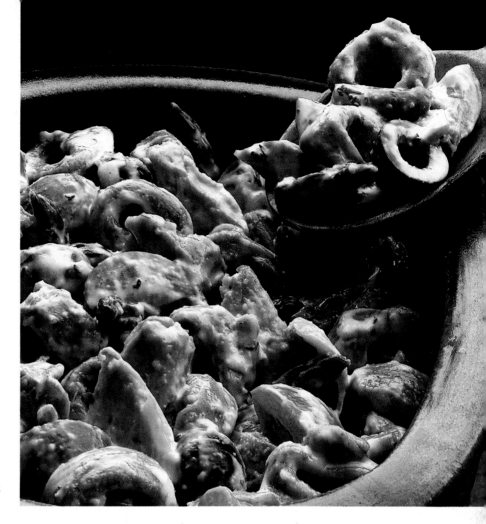

Creamy Tortellini & Salmon Salad ▲

Dressing:
½ cup mayonnaise
⅓ cup half-and-half
⅓ cup grated Parmesan cheese
1 teaspoon dried parsley flakes
¼ teaspoon dried thyme leaves
⅛ teaspoon garlic powder
⅛ teaspoon pepper

1 pkg. (6 oz.) uncooked spinach tortellini

¼ lb. fresh asparagus, cut into ½-inch pieces
1 tablespoon water
1 jar (6 oz.) marinated artichoke hearts, drained and cut up
½ cup quartered cherry tomatoes
½ cup pitted black olives, cut in half
1 can (6¾ oz.) skinless, boneless salmon, drained

4 to 6 servings

In small mixing bowl, combine all dressing ingredients. Mix well. Set aside. Prepare tortellini as directed on package. Rinse with cold water. Drain. Place in large mixing bowl. Set aside.

In 1-quart casserole, combine asparagus and water. Cover. Microwave at High for 1 to 2 minutes, or until asparagus is very hot and color brightens. Rinse with cold water. Drain. Add to cooked tortellini with dressing and remaining ingredients. Toss gently to coat. Cover and chill for 2 to 3 hours before serving.

Creamy Tortellini & Ham Salad: Follow recipe above, except substitute ⅔ cup fully cooked cubed ham (½-inch cubes) for salmon.

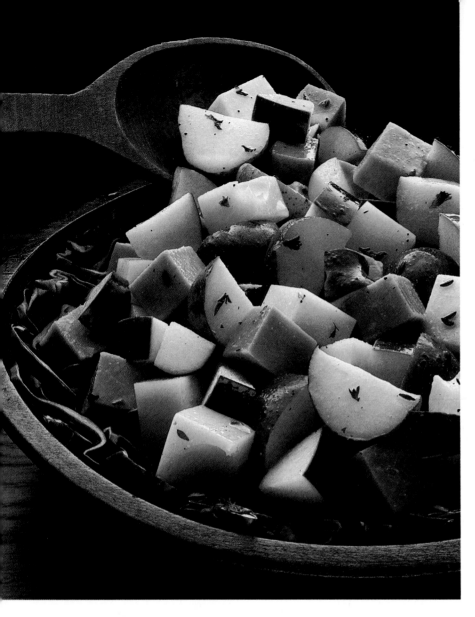

Bavarian Ham & Potato Salad

Dressing:

⅔ cup vegetable oil
⅓ cup cider vinegar
2 teaspoons packed brown
    sugar
½ teaspoon dried parsley flakes
½ teaspoon caraway seed
½ teaspoon dry mustard
¼ teaspoon salt
⅛ teaspoon pepper

1 lb. new potatoes
1 small apple
½ lb. fully cooked ham, cut into
    bite-size pieces
¼ lb. Swiss cheese, cut into
    bite-size pieces
4 cups shredded red cabbage

4 servings

How to Microwave Bavarian Ham & Potato Salad

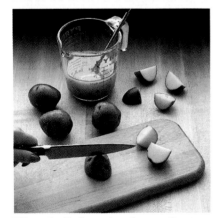

Blend all dressing ingredients in 2-cup measure. Set aside. Cut largest potatoes into quarters. Cut smaller potatoes in half. Place in 1½-quart casserole.

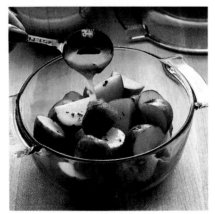

Stir dressing. Spoon 3 tablespoons dressing over potatoes. Stir to coat. Cover. Microwave at High for 8 to 10 minutes, or until potatoes are tender, stirring once. Chill for at least 2 hours.

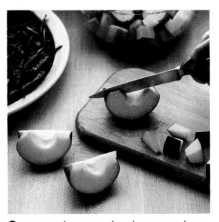

Core and coarsely chop apple. In medium mixing bowl, combine apple, potatoes, ham and cheese. Add remaining dressing. Stir to coat. Spread cabbage on serving platter or in shallow bowl. Top with potato salad.

7-Layer Beef Salad ▶

1 lb. boneless beef sirloin
   steak, about 1 inch thick
1 tablespoon Worcestershire
   sauce
¼ teaspoon onion powder
⅛ teaspoon garlic powder
½ teaspoon coarsely ground
   pepper
4 oz. fresh pea pods
2 tablespoons water
4 cups torn fresh spinach
   leaves or leaf lettuce
1 cup cherry tomato halves
¾ cup fresh sliced mushrooms
½ cup sliced red onion
½ cup sour cream
¼ cup mayonnaise
2 teaspoons white wine vinegar
¼ teaspoon salt
¼ cup crumbled blue cheese
1 tablespoon snipped fresh
   parsley

6 to 8 servings

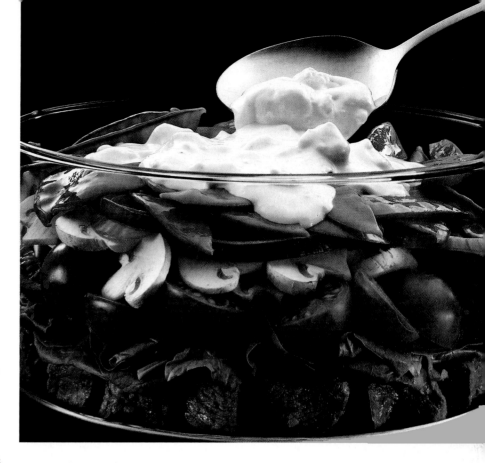

Pierce sirloin thoroughly with fork. Place on roasting rack. Set aside. In small bowl, combine Worcestershire sauce and onion and garlic powders. Mix well. Brush on all surfaces of sirloin. Sprinkle top of sirloin with pepper. Microwave at 70% (Medium High) for 6 to 11 minutes, or until medium rare, rotating rack once. Cool slightly. Cut into ½-inch cubes. Place in large mixing bowl. Set aside.

In 1-quart casserole, combine pea pods and water. Cover. Microwave at High for 1 to 2 minutes, or until pea pods are very hot and color brightens. Rinse with cold water. Drain. Set aside. To assemble salad, layer spinach leaves over beef. Continue layering tomato halves, mushrooms, onion, and pea pods. Set aside.

In 2-cup measure, combine sour cream, mayonnaise, vinegar and salt. Mix well. Stir in blue cheese. Pour over salad. Spread evenly. Sprinkle with parsley. Cover and chill for at least 3 hours. Toss salad before serving.

Tossed Garden Salad with Sirloin

1 lb. boneless beef sirloin
   steak, about 1 inch thick
1 small onion, thinly sliced
1 clove garlic, cut into quarters
2 tablespoons red wine vinegar
1 tablespoon vegetable oil
2 teaspoons Worcestershire
   sauce
¼ teaspoon dried marjoram
   leaves
1 cup fresh cauliflowerets
⅓ cup sliced carrot (¼-inch
   slices)

2 tablespoons water
4 cups torn romaine lettuce
⅓ cup julienne zucchini
   (1½ × ¼-inch strips)
½ small red pepper, cut into
   ¼-inch strips

Dressing:
¼ cup vegetable oil
1 tablespoon plus 1 teaspoon
   red wine vinegar
¼ teaspoon garlic salt
⅛ teaspoon pepper

6 to 8 servings

In large plastic food-storage bag, combine steak, onion and garlic. Set aside. In 1-cup measure, blend vinegar, oil, Worcestershire sauce and marjoram. Add to steak mixture. Secure bag. Refrigerate for at least 2 hours.

Remove steak from marinade, discarding marinade. On roasting rack, microwave steak at 70% (Medium High) for 6 to 11 minutes, or just until medium rare, rotating rack once. Chill for at least 1 hour. Slice into thin strips and place in large mixing bowl. Set aside.

In 1-quart casserole, combine cauliflower, carrot and water. Cover. Microwave at High for 2 to 3 minutes, or just until vegetables are tender-crisp, stirring once. Rinse under cold water. Drain. Add cauliflower, carrot, lettuce, zucchini and red pepper to sirloin strips. Set aside. Blend all dressing ingredients in 1-cup measure. Pour over salad and toss to coat. Sprinkle with croutons, if desired. Serve immediately.

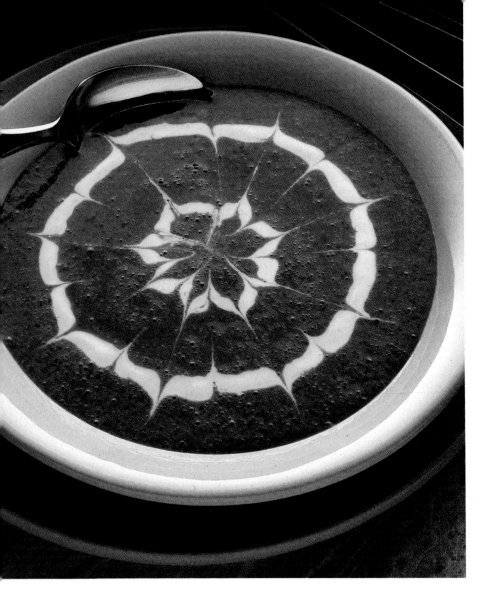

Cold Cherry Soup

2 cups frozen pitted dark sweet cherries
⅓ cup sugar
⅛ teaspoon ground cinnamon
¼ cup white wine
1 cup buttermilk
1 tablespoon sour cream

4 to 6 servings

Cold Peach Soup: Follow recipe above, except substitute 2 cups frozen sliced peaches for cherries. Microwave at High for 10 to 15 minutes, or until peaches are tender, stirring once or twice.

How to Microwave Cold Cherry Soup

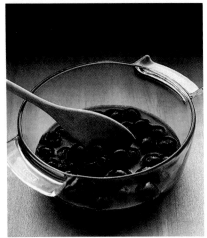

Combine all ingredients, except buttermilk and sour cream, in 1½-quart casserole. Mix well. Microwave at High for 7 to 10 minutes, or until mixture bubbles and sugar dissolves, stirring once.

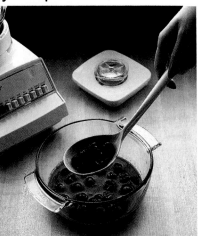

Remove cherries with slotted spoon, reserving cooking liquid. In blender or food processor, process cherries until smooth. Blend in cooking liquid and buttermilk. Chill for at least 1 hour.

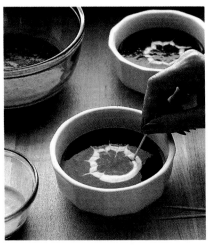

Blend 1 teaspoon chilled soup and the sour cream in small bowl. Spoon soup into individual dishes. Top each serving with sour cream mixture. Using wooden pick, make a swirl design in each sour cream topping.

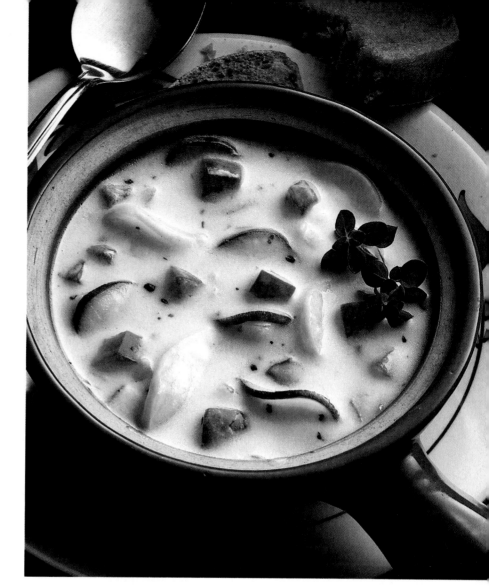

Creamy Italian ▶ Summer Squash Soup

- ¼ cup chopped onion
- 2 tablespoons olive or vegetable oil
- 1 clove garlic, minced
- ½ teaspoon Italian seasoning
- 1 medium zucchini, thinly sliced
- 1 medium summer squash, thinly sliced
- ¼ cup all-purpose flour
- ½ teaspoon salt
- ⅛ teaspoon pepper
- 1½ cups milk
- ¾ cup ready-to-serve chicken broth
- ½ cup seeded chopped tomato

4 servings

In 2-quart casserole, combine onion, oil, garlic and Italian seasoning. Cover. Microwave at High for 3 to 3½ minutes, or until onion is tender. Stir in zucchini and summer squash. Re-cover. Microwave at High for 6 to 9 minutes, or until squash is very tender, stirring 2 or 3 times.

Sprinkle flour, salt and pepper over squash. Stir to coat. Blend in milk and chicken broth until smooth. Microwave at High for 7½ to 11 minutes, or until mixture thickens and bubbles around edges, stirring 2 or 3 times. Stir in tomato. Let stand for 3 minutes. Sprinkle with grated Parmesan cheese before serving, if desired.

Ginger Carrot Soup

- 2 cups sliced carrots (½-inch slices)
- 1 cup peeled cubed potato (¾-inch cubes)
- 1 small onion, chopped
- ½ cup water
- 3 tablespoons butter or margarine
- 2 tablespoons soy sauce
- 1 teaspoon instant chicken bouillon granules
- 1 teaspoon packed brown sugar
- 1 teaspoon grated fresh gingerroot
- ½ teaspoon ground coriander
- 1¼ cups milk
  Yogurt or sour cream
  Fresh parsley sprigs

4 servings

In 1½-quart casserole, combine all ingredients except milk, yogurt and parsley. Cover. Microwave at High for 17 to 22 minutes, or until vegetables are very tender, stirring once or twice. Let stand, covered, for 10 minutes.

Place vegetable mixture in food processor or blender. Process until smooth. Return to casserole. Blend in milk. Cover. Microwave at High for 2 to 3 minutes, or until soup is hot. Garnish each serving with yogurt and a fresh parsley sprig, if desired. Soup may be served chilled.

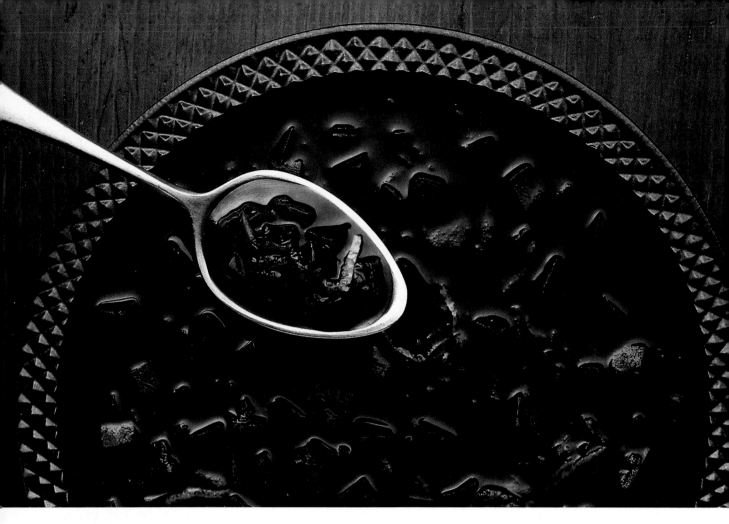

Creamy Leek Soup

- 1 medium leek
- 3 tablespoons butter or margarine
- 1½ cups milk
- 1 can (10¾ oz.) condensed cream of potato soup
- 1 teaspoon instant chicken bouillon granules
- ⅛ teaspoon pepper
  Dash ground nutmeg

4 servings

Trim ends and cut leek in half lengthwise. Rinse under cold water to remove dirt. Slice leek crosswise into ½-inch pieces. In 2-quart casserole, place leek slices and butter. Cover. Microwave at High for 8 to 10 minutes, or until leeks are tender, stirring 2 or 3 times.

Add milk, potato soup, chicken bouillon granules and pepper. Mix well. Re-cover. Microwave at High for 4 to 7 minutes, or until soup is hot, stirring once or twice. Before serving, sprinkle with nutmeg.

Creamy Leek and Shrimp Soup: Follow recipe above, except add 1 can (4¼ oz.) large canned shrimp, rinsed and drained, with milk and remaining ingredients.

Beet Soup ▲

- ½ cup finely shredded apple
- ¼ cup finely chopped onion
- 1 tablespoon butter or margarine
- 1 tablespoon cornstarch
- ½ teaspoon grated orange peel (optional)
- ⅛ teaspoon ground cloves
- 1 can (14½ oz.) ready-to-serve beef broth
- 1 can (16 oz.) diced beets, rinsed and drained

4 servings

In 1½-quart casserole, combine apple, onion and butter. Cover. Microwave at High for 3 to 5 minutes, or until onion is tender, stirring once. Stir in cornstarch, orange peel and cloves. Blend in beef broth. Microwave, uncovered, at High for 11 to 18 minutes, or until mixture is thickened and slightly translucent, stirring 2 or 3 times. Stir in beets. Cover. Let stand for 2 minutes.

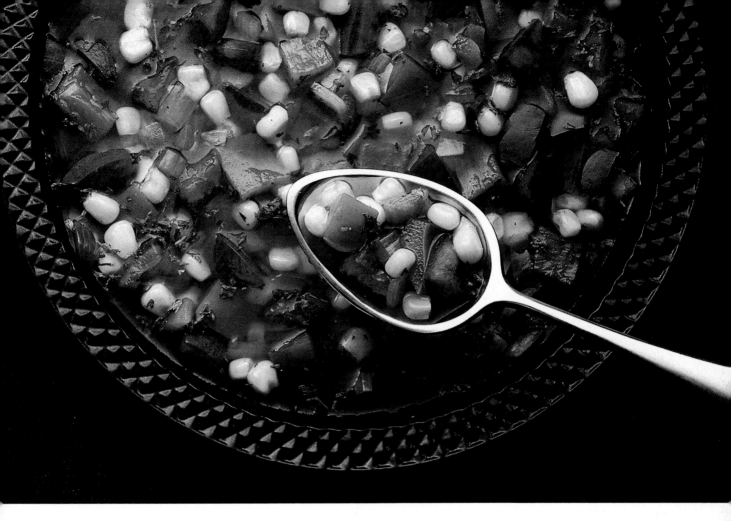

Avocado Soup

2 cans (14½ oz. each) ready-
   to-serve chicken broth
½ cup half-and-half
½ teaspoon salt
⅛ teaspoon ground cumin
2 avocados, peeled and
   seeded
2 tablespoons chopped onion
2 tablespoons lime juice

4 to 6 servings

In 2-quart casserole, combine
broth, half-and-half, salt and
cumin. Cover. Microwave at High
for 5 to 9 minutes, or just until
mixture is hot, stirring once. In
food processor or blender, place
avocados, onion and lime juice.
Process until smooth. Blend a
small amount of avocado mixture
into hot broth mixture. Add remaining avocado mixture and
blend with whisk until smooth.
Serve immediately. Garnish each
serving with avocado and lime
slices, if desired.

Mexican Corn Chowder ▲

½ cup chopped onion
⅓ cup chopped green pepper
2 tablespoons butter or
   margarine
1 clove garlic, minced
¼ teaspoon ground cumin
⅛ teaspoon chili powder
1 can (10¾ oz.) condensed
   chicken broth
1 cup water
1 pkg. (10 oz.) frozen corn
1 medium tomato, seeded and
   chopped
2 tablespoons canned
   chopped green chilies
1 teaspoon dried parsley flakes
½ teaspoon salt

4 servings

In 2-quart casserole, combine onion, green pepper, butter, garlic, cumin
and chili powder. Cover. Microwave at High for 5 to 7 minutes, or until
vegetables are tender, stirring once or twice. Add remaining ingredients.
Re-cover. Microwave at High for 8 to 12 minutes, or until soup is hot,
stirring once or twice.

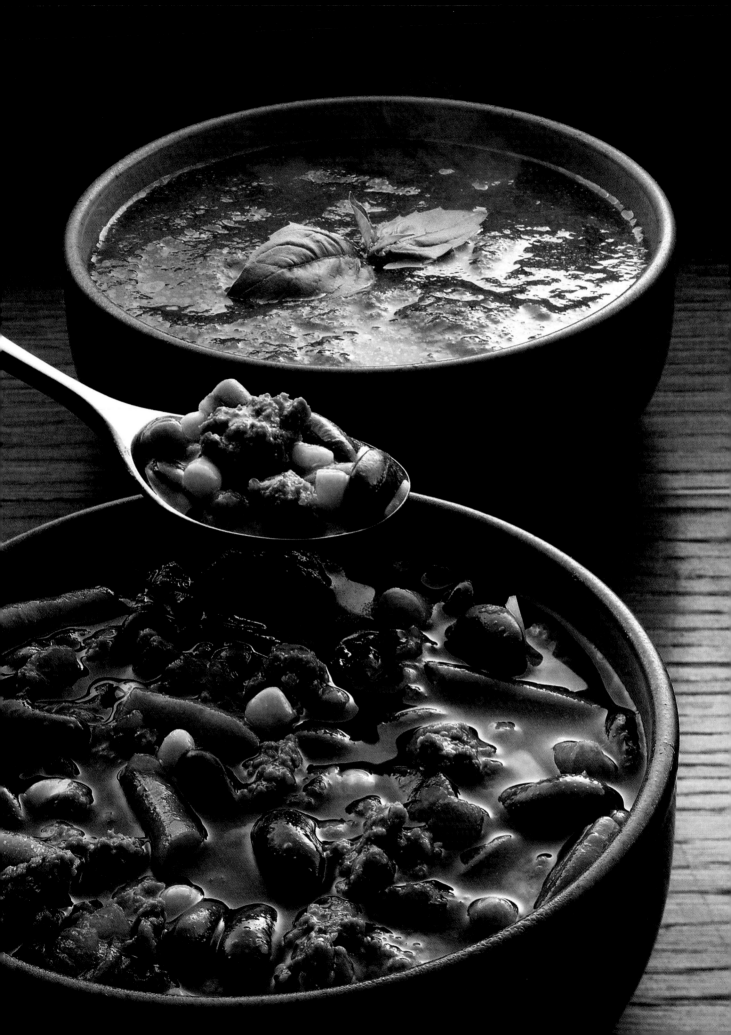

◄ Fresh Tomato Basil Soup

4 medium tomatoes (about 2 lbs.)
4 cups hot water
4 cups ice water
2 tablespoons finely chopped shallot
1 tablespoon snipped fresh basil
2 teaspoons snipped fresh parsley

1 tablespoon olive oil
2 cups tomato juice
2 teaspoons sugar
1 teaspoon instant beef bouillon granules
¾ teaspoon salt
⅛ teaspoon pepper

4 to 6 servings

Using sharp knife, cut a crossmark on bottom of each tomato. Place hot water in 2-quart casserole. Microwave at High for 6 to 11 minutes, or until boiling, covered. Add tomatoes. Let stand for 1½ minutes.

In medium mixing bowl, immerse tomatoes briefly in ice water. Core and peel. Cut in half; remove and discard seeds. In food processor or blender, process tomatoes until smooth. Set aside.

In 2-quart casserole, combine shallot, basil, parsley and olive oil. Cover. Microwave at High for 1½ to 2 minutes, or until shallot is tender. Stir in tomato mixture and remaining ingredients. Re-cover. Microwave at High for 8 to 11 minutes, or until soup is hot, stirring once. Serve hot or chilled.

Easy Tomato Basil Soup: Follow recipe above, except substitute 1 can (15 oz.) tomato purée and 2½ cups tomato juice for fresh tomatoes. Substitute 1 teaspoon each of dried basil leaves and dried parsley flakes for fresh basil and parsley.

◄ Vegetable-Beef Soup

½ lb. ground beef
¼ cup chopped onion
2 cups hot water
1 can (16 oz.) whole tomatoes, drained and cut up
½ cup frozen cut green beans
2 teaspoons instant beef bouillon granules
2 teaspoons instant chicken bouillon granules

½ teaspoon dried marjoram leaves
¼ teaspoon salt
1 small bay leaf
1 can (15 oz.) kidney beans, drained
½ cup frozen corn
½ cup frozen peas

6 to 8 servings

Crumble beef into 2-quart casserole. Add onion. Cover. Microwave at High for 3 to 5 minutes, or until meat is no longer pink, stirring once. Stir in water, tomatoes, green beans, beef and chicken bouillon granules, marjoram, salt and bay leaf. Re-cover. Microwave at High for 5 to 6 minutes, or until mixture is hot.

Microwave mixture at 70% (Medium High) for 15 to 20 minutes longer, or just until beans are tender, stirring once or twice. Stir in remaining ingredients. Re-cover. Microwave at 70% (Medium High) for 5 minutes. Let stand, covered, for 5 minutes.

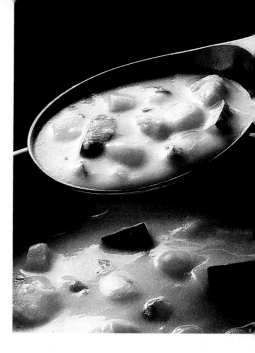

Vegetable Clam Chowder ▲

1 cup chopped zucchini
⅓ cup chopped onion
2 tablespoons butter or margarine
1 tablespoon snipped fresh parsley
½ teaspoon dried marjoram leaves
¼ cup all-purpose flour
2 teaspoons instant chicken bouillon granules
⅛ teaspoon pepper
2 cups milk
1 can (6½ oz.) minced clams, drained, reserve juice
1 can (17 oz.) corn, drained

4 servings

In 2-quart casserole, combine zucchini, onion, butter, parsley and marjoram. Cover. Microwave at High for 4 to 7 minutes, or until vegetables are tender, stirring once. Sprinkle flour, chicken bouillon granules and pepper over vegetables. Stir to coat.

Blend in milk and reserved clam juice. Microwave at High for 7 to 11 minutes, or until mixture thickens and bubbles around edges, stirring 2 or 3 times. Stir in clams and corn. Microwave for 2 to 3 minutes, or until chowder is hot.

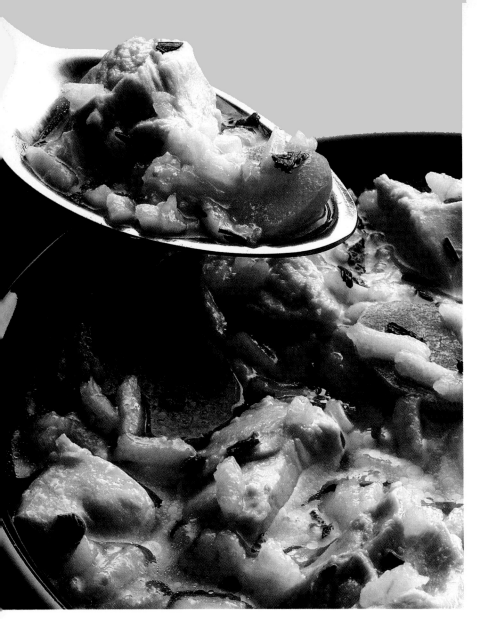

Breast of Chicken with Rice Soup ▲

1 can (14½ oz.) ready-to-serve
   chicken broth
⅓ cup diagonally sliced carrot
   (⅛ inch thick)
¼ teaspoon dried tarragon
   leaves

1 boneless whole chicken
   breast (10 to 12 oz.), skin
   removed, cut into 1-inch
   pieces
½ cup instant rice
⅔ cup torn fresh spinach leaves
   (optional)

4 servings

In 1½-quart casserole, combine chicken broth, carrot and tarragon. Cover. Microwave at High for 5 to 8 minutes, or just until broth is boiling. Add chicken pieces and rice. Re-cover. Microwave at High for 5 to 7 minutes, or until chicken is no longer pink. Stir in spinach. Re-cover. Let stand for 5 minutes.

Black Bean Soup

¾ cup chopped onion
½ cup chopped green pepper
1 clove garlic, minced
1 tablespoon snipped fresh
   parsley
¼ teaspoon dried oregano
   leaves
½ teaspoon ground cumin
⅛ teaspoon dried thyme leaves
   Dash cayenne
2 tablespoons olive oil
1 can (10¾ oz.) condensed
   chicken broth
¾ cup water
¾ cup cubed fully cooked ham
   (½-inch cubes)
1 can (8 oz.) whole tomatoes,
   cut up
1 tablespoon red wine vinegar
2 cans (15 oz. each) black
   beans

6 to 8 servings

In 2-quart casserole, combine onion, green pepper, garlic, parsley, oregano, cumin, thyme, cayenne and oil. Cover. Microwave at High for 3½ to 5½ minutes, or until onion is tender, stirring once. Stir in remaining ingredients, except black beans. Re-cover. Microwave at High for 7 to 12 minutes, or until mixture is hot and bubbly, stirring once. Stir in beans. Re-cover. Microwave at High for 2 to 3 minutes, or until soup is hot. Garnish with sliced green onion, if desired.

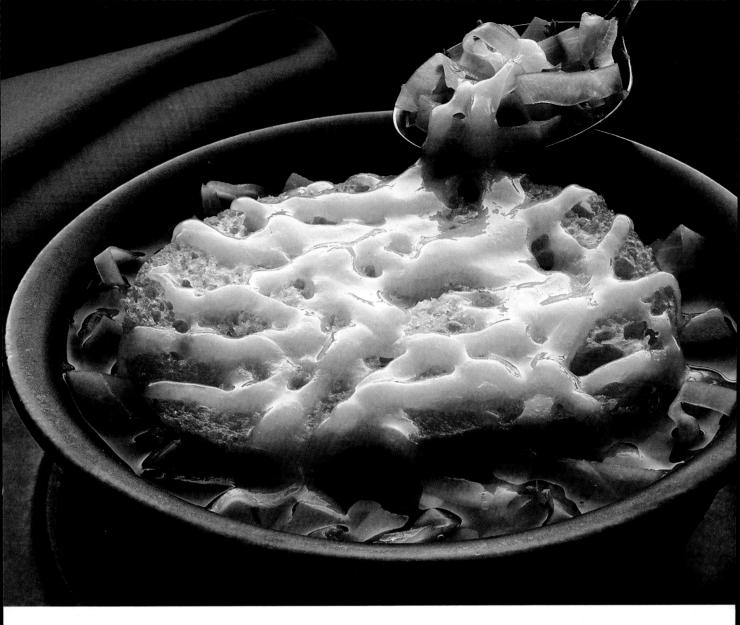

St. Pat's Day Soup

- ⅓ cup chopped carrot
- ⅓ cup chopped onion
- 2 tablespoons butter or margarine
- 2 teaspoons snipped fresh parsley
- ¼ teaspoon caraway seed
  Dash pepper
- 3 cups water
- 2 cups thinly sliced cabbage
- 1½ teaspoons instant beef bouillon granules
- 1½ teaspoons instant chicken bouillon granules
- 4 slices French bread (½ inch thick), toasted
- ½ cup shredded Swiss cheese
  Paprika

4 servings

In 2-quart casserole, combine carrot, onion, butter, parsley, caraway seed and pepper. Cover. Microwave at High for 4 to 5 minutes, or until vegetables are tender, stirring once. Stir in water, cabbage, and beef and chicken bouillon granules. Re-cover. Microwave at High for 12 to 17 minutes, or until cabbage is tender, stirring once or twice.

Divide soup evenly among four 15-oz. bowls. Top each serving with bread. Top each bread slice with 1 tablespoon cheese. Sprinkle with paprika. Microwave at High for 3 to 5 minutes, or until cheese melts, rearranging bowls once.

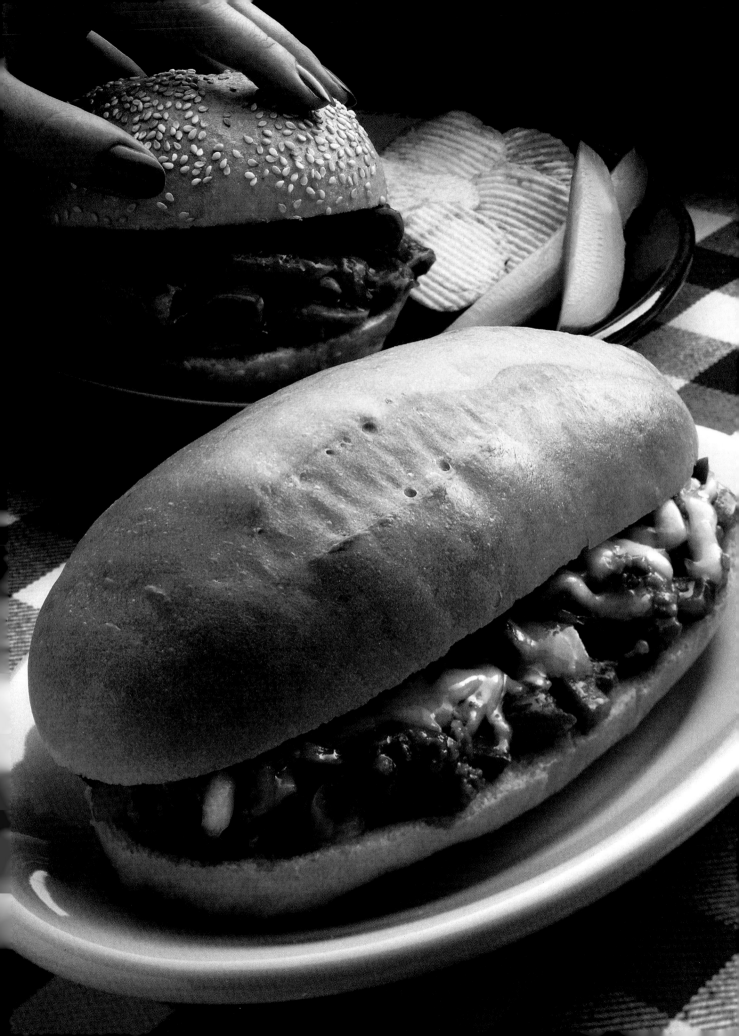

◄ Hot Barbecue Sandwiches

2½- lb. boneless pork loin roast	1 can (4 oz.) chopped green chilies
1½ teaspoons crushed red pepper flakes, divided	1 medium onion, thinly sliced
½ teaspoon dried oregano leaves	⅓ cup ready-to-serve chicken broth
¼ teaspoon dried thyme leaves	2 cups barbecue sauce Sandwich rolls

10 to 12 servings

Place pork roast in nylon cooking bag. Sprinkle evenly with 1 teaspoon red pepper flakes, the oregano and thyme. Top with chilies, onion and chicken broth. Secure bag loosely with nylon tie or string. Place in 9-inch square baking dish.

Microwave roast at High for 5 minutes. Rotate dish. Microwave at 70% (Medium High) for 35 to 40 minutes longer, or until internal temperature in center reaches 165°F, turning bag over once. Let bag stand, closed, for 10 minutes. Remove roast and set aside to cool slightly. Strain and discard cooking liquid, reserving onion mixture. Set aside.

Trim and discard fat and any gristle from roast. Shred roast, or shave on meat slicer. Set aside.

In medium mixing bowl, combine onion mixture, barbecue sauce and the remaining ½ teaspoon red pepper flakes. Microwave at High for 2 to 3 minutes, or until hot. Add shredded pork. Mix well. Microwave at High for 4 to 6 minutes, or until hot. Serve on sandwich rolls.

◄ Italian Sloppy Subs

½ lb. ground Italian sausage	½ teaspoon Italian seasoning
½ cup coarsely chopped onion	¼ cup butter or margarine
½ cup coarsely chopped green pepper	¼ teaspoon garlic powder
1 can (8 oz.) whole tomatoes, drained and cut up	4 French rolls (6 to 8-inch), split
¼ cup catsup	1 cup shredded mozzarella cheese

4 servings

In 1-quart casserole, combine sausage, onion and green pepper. Cover. Microwave at High for 4 to 5 minutes, or until meat is no longer pink, stirring several times to break apart. Drain. Add tomatoes, catsup and Italian seasoning. Microwave at High for 2 to 4 minutes, or until mixture is hot and flavors are blended, stirring once. Set aside.

In small bowl, microwave butter and garlic powder at High for 1¼ to 1½ minutes, or until butter melts. Brush on insides of rolls. Place rolls cut-side-up under conventional broiler, 2 to 3 inches from heat. Broil until golden brown.

Arrange bottom halves of rolls on paper-towel-lined plate. Top each with one-fourth of meat mixture. Sprinkle evenly with cheese. Microwave at 70% (Medium High) for 2 to 4 minutes, or until cheese melts. Add tops of rolls. Serve hot.

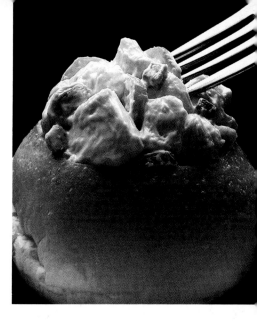

Chicken Cashew ▲ Sandwiches

Marinade:

¼ cup pineapple juice
½ teaspoon ground coriander
⅛ teaspoon ground ginger

1 boneless whole chicken breast (10 to 12 oz.), skin removed, cut into ¾-inch pieces
½ cup coarsely chopped cashews
½ cup sliced celery
⅓ cup finely chopped onion
¼ cup finely chopped red or green pepper
2 tablespoons mayonnaise
2 tablespoons sour cream
2 tablespoons drained crushed pineapple (optional)
¼ teaspoon salt
⅛ teaspoon ground coriander
Hard rolls or sliced bread

2 to 4 servings

In 1-quart casserole, mix all marinade ingredients. Add chicken pieces and stir to coat. Cover. Refrigerate for at least 1 hour, stirring once. Microwave at High for 3½ to 6 minutes, or until chicken is no longer pink, stirring once. Drain.

Add remaining ingredients, except rolls. Mix well. Chill, if desired. Spoon into hollowed-out rolls or use as sandwich filling with bread slices.

Mexican Patty Melts ▼

- 1 lb. ground beef
- 2 tablespoons salsa
- 2 tablespoons sliced green onion
- ½ teaspoon chili powder
- ¼ teaspoon garlic salt
- ¼ teaspoon ground cumin
- 4 slices (¾ oz. each) Monterey Jack or Colby cheese
- 4 hamburger buns

4 sandwiches

In medium mixing bowl, combine ground beef, salsa, onion, chili powder, garlic salt and cumin. Mix well. Shape into 4 patties, about ½ inch thick. Arrange on roasting rack. Microwave at High for 4½ to 7½ minutes, or until meat is firm and no longer pink, rearranging and turning over once. Top each patty with cheese. Cover with wax paper and let stand for 2 to 3 minutes. Serve in buns. Garnish with leaf lettuce, if desired.

Mock Gyros

Sauce:

- ⅓ cup plain yogurt
- 2 tablespoons sour cream
- 2 tablespoons finely chopped cucumber
- ½ teaspoon grated lemon peel
- ¼ teaspoon dried mint flakes
- ¼ teaspoon sugar
- ⅛ teaspoon salt

Meat mixture:

- ½ lb. ground beef
- ½ lb. ground lamb
- 1 teaspoon dried oregano leaves
- ½ teaspoon salt
- ¼ teaspoon ground cinnamon
- ⅛ teaspoon dried thyme leaves
- ⅛ teaspoon garlic powder
- 4 pitas (6-inch)

4 sandwiches

Blend sauce ingredients in small mixing bowl. Cover. Chill for at least 30 minutes. In 1-quart casserole, combine beef, lamb, oregano, salt, cinnamon, thyme and garlic powder. Mix well. Microwave at High for 4 to 7 minutes, or until meat is no longer pink, stirring once. Drain. Spoon into pitas. Add shredded lettuce, if desired. Serve with sauce.

Variation: Prepare and chill sauce as directed. Combine meat and seasonings as directed. Mix well. Form into 4 patties, about ½ inch thick. Arrange on roasting rack. Microwave at High for 3½ to 5½ minutes, or until meat is firm and no longer pink, rearranging and turning patties over once. Serve in hamburger buns with sauce.

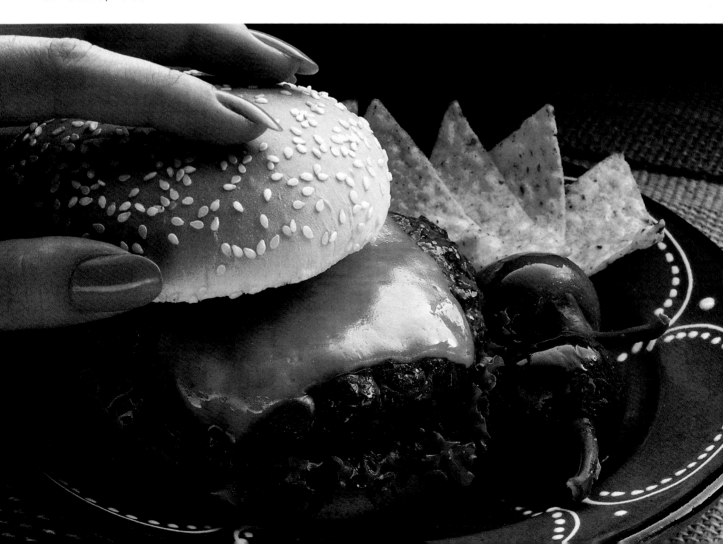

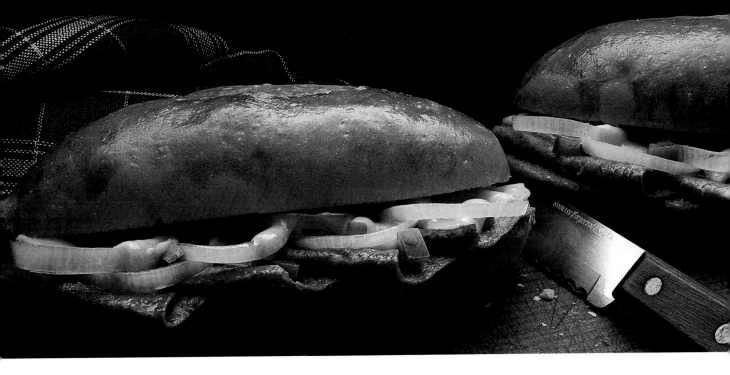

Philly Beef Sandwiches

1 medium green pepper,
   coarsely chopped
1 medium onion, sliced
2 tablespoons butter or
   margarine
4 frozen beef sandwich steaks
   (2 oz. each)
4 French rolls (6 to 8-inch), split
6 slices (¾ oz. each)
   pasteurized process
   American cheese, cut
   in half

4 sandwiches

How to Microwave Philly Beef Sandwiches

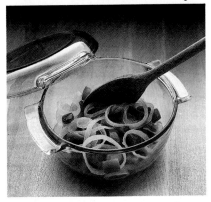

Combine green pepper, onion and butter in 1-quart casserole. Cover. Microwave at High for 3 to 4 minutes, or until vegetables are tender-crisp, stirring once. Set aside.

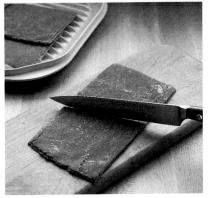

Cut frozen steaks in half. Place halves on roasting rack, overlapping if necessary. Microwave at High for 3 to 4½ minutes, or until meat is no longer pink, rearranging once.

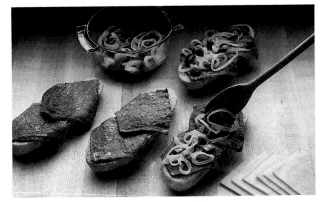

Place 2 pieces of meat on each of 4 French roll halves. Top evenly with onion mixture and cheese.

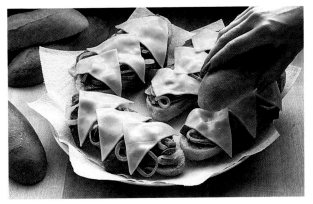

Layer 2 paper towels on 12-inch round platter. Arrange open face sandwiches on platter. Microwave at High for 1¼ to 1¾ minutes, or until cheese melts. Add top halves of rolls to serve.

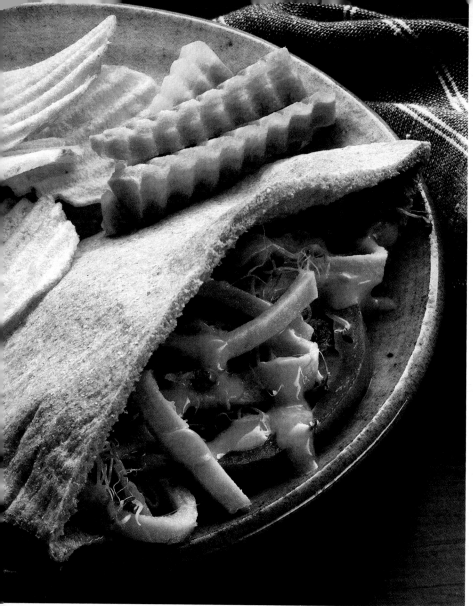

Turkey Club Pitas ◀

4 slices bacon
1 cup thin strips smoked turkey breast (3 to 4 oz.)
½ cup shredded Cheddar cheese
½ cup alfalfa sprouts
2 tablespoons finely chopped onion
2 pitas (6-inch), cut in half
   Mayonnaise
   Prepared mustard
4 thin slices tomato

4 sandwiches

Arrange bacon slices on roasting rack. Cover with paper towel. Microwave at High for 3 to 6 minutes, or until brown and crisp. Cool slightly. Crumble. In small mixing bowl, combine bacon, turkey, cheese, sprouts and onion. Mix well. Spread insides of pitas with mayonnaise and mustard. Place 1 tomato slice inside each pita. Place one-fourth of turkey mixture inside each pita.

Arrange pocket sandwiches on paper-towel-lined plate. Microwave at 70% (Medium High) for 2½ to 5 minutes, or just until cheese begins to melt, rotating plate once or twice.

Salmon Smokies ▶

1 can (6¾ oz.) skinless, boneless salmon, drained
2 tablespoons mayonnaise
1 tablespoon sliced pimiento, drained
1 tablespoon sliced green onion
½ teaspoon lemon juice
   Dash pepper
2 English muffins, split and toasted
4 thin green pepper rings
4 slices (½ oz. each) smoked sharp Cheddar cheese

4 sandwiches

In small mixing bowl, combine salmon, mayonnaise, pimiento, onion, lemon juice and pepper. Mix well. Spread one-fourth of salmon mixture on each split English muffin. Top with green pepper ring and cheese slice. Place on paper-towel-lined plate. Microwave at 70% (Medium High) for 3 to 4½ minutes, or until cheese melts, rotating plate once.

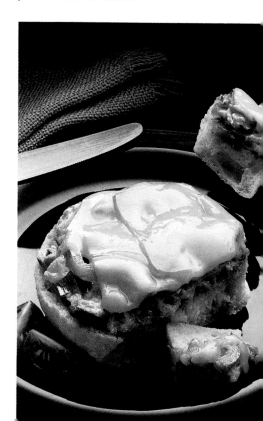

Summer Vegie Melt ▶

¼ cup butter or margarine
1½ teaspoons lemon juice
1 teaspoon Dijon mustard
¼ teaspoon dried marjoram
    leaves
1 cup small fresh broccoli
    flowerets
8 small fresh asparagus
    spears, trimmed and cut
    in half
2 Kaiser rolls, split
½ cup torn fresh spinach
    leaves
½ cup thinly sliced fresh
    mushrooms
⅓ cup thinly sliced zucchini or
    summer squash
⅓ cup alfalfa sprouts
2 thin red or green pepper
    rings
2 slices (1 oz. each)
    Provolone cheese

2 sandwiches

In 1-cup measure, combine butter, lemon juice, mustard and marjoram. Microwave at High for 1¼ to 1¾ minutes, or until butter melts. Stir to blend. Place broccoli in small mixing bowl. Drizzle with 1 tablespoon butter mixture. Cover with plastic wrap. Microwave at High for 1 to 1¾ minutes, or until broccoli is very hot and color brightens. Uncover and set aside.

Place asparagus on small plate. Drizzle with 2 teaspoons butter mixture. Cover with plastic wrap. Microwave at High for 45 seconds to 1¼ minutes, or until asparagus is very hot and color brightens. Set aside.

Brush cut side of each roll half with remaining butter mixture. Arrange bottom halves of rolls on paper-towel-lined plate. Layer vegetables evenly on roll halves. Top each serving with slice of cheese. Microwave at 70% (Medium High) for 2¾ to 3½ minutes, or until cheese melts, rotating plate once. Top with remaining roll halves.

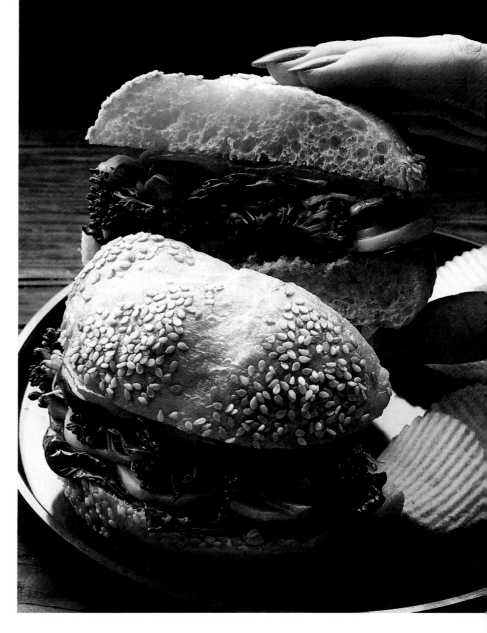

Triple-Cheese Sandwiches

1 pkg. (3 oz.) cream cheese
1 tablespoon mayonnaise
1 tablespoon sliced green onion
    Prepared mustard (optional)
8 slices rye bread, toasted

4 slices (¾ oz. each) Colby
    cheese
4 slices (¾ oz. each) Monterey
    Jack cheese
    Cherry tomatoes, cut in half
    (optional)

4 sandwiches

In small mixing bowl, microwave cream cheese at High for 15 to 30 seconds, or until softened. Add mayonnaise and onion. Mix well. Spread mustard on one side of each slice of bread. Spread cream cheese mixture evenly over mustard. Layer 4 slices of bread with 1 slice each of Colby and Monterey Jack cheeses. Top with remaining slices of bread.

On paper-towel-lined plate, microwave sandwiches at 70% (Medium High) for 2 to 3½ minutes, or until cheeses melt, rotating once or twice. Place cherry tomato halves on wooden picks and garnish sandwich tops.

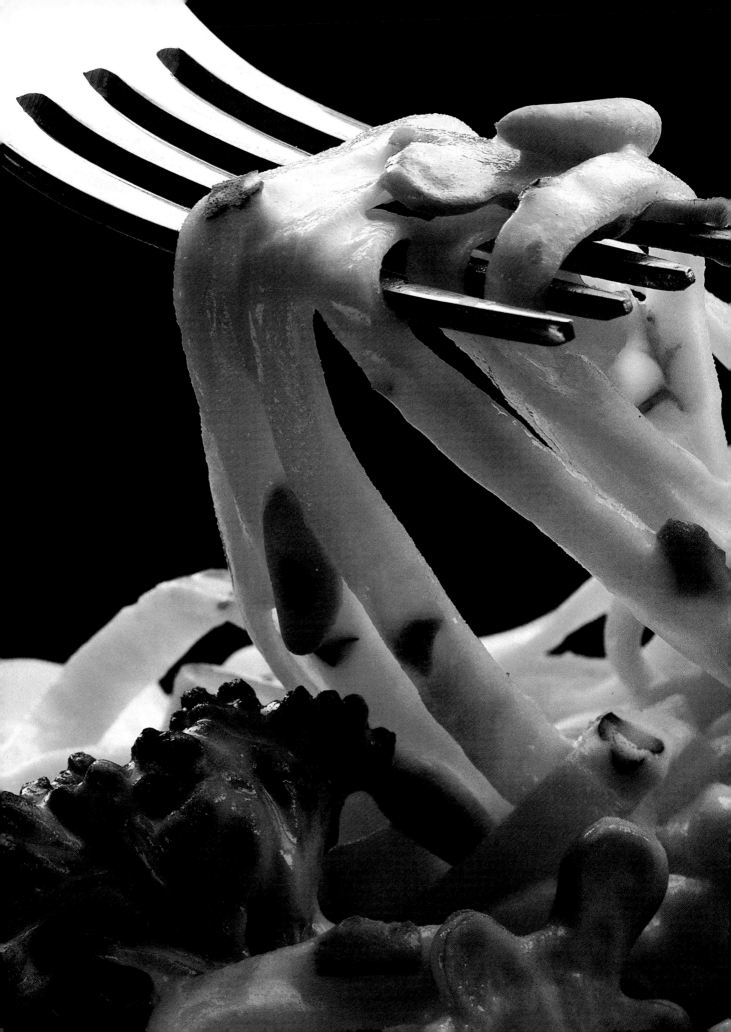

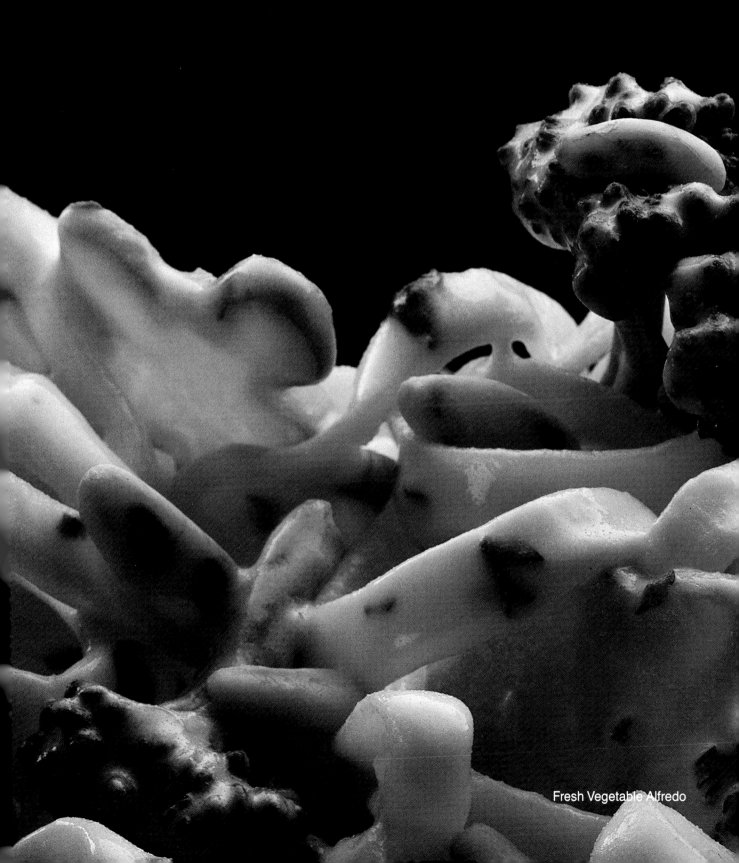

Meatless Entrées

Fresh Vegetable Alfredo

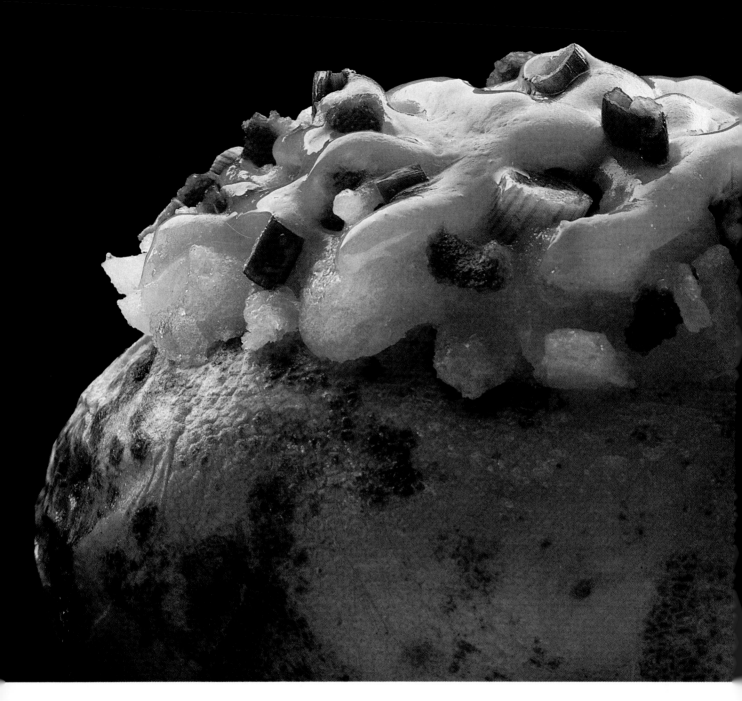

Stuffed Cheese Potatoes ▲

4   medium baking potatoes
    (8 to 10 oz. each)
1½ cups shredded Cheddar
    cheese, divided
¼   cup butter or margarine
½   cup milk
⅓   cup bacon-flavored bits
    (optional)
¼   cup sliced green onions
½   teaspoon salt
½   teaspoon dry mustard
¼   teaspoon pepper

4 servings

Pierce potatoes with fork. Arrange in circle on paper towel in microwave oven. Microwave at High for 10 to 16 minutes, or just until tender, turning over and rearranging once. Let stand for 5 minutes. Cut a thin slice from top of each potato. Scoop out pulp, leaving about ¼-inch shell. Set shells aside.

Place pulp in medium mixing bowl. Add 1 cup cheese, the butter, milk, bacon-flavored bits, onion, salt, dry mustard and pepper. Beat at medium speed of an electric mixer until blended. Spoon mixture evenly into potato shells. Arrange potatoes on platter. Sprinkle with remaining ½ cup cheese. Microwave at High for 5 to 10 minutes, or until potatoes are hot and cheese is melted, rotating platter once.

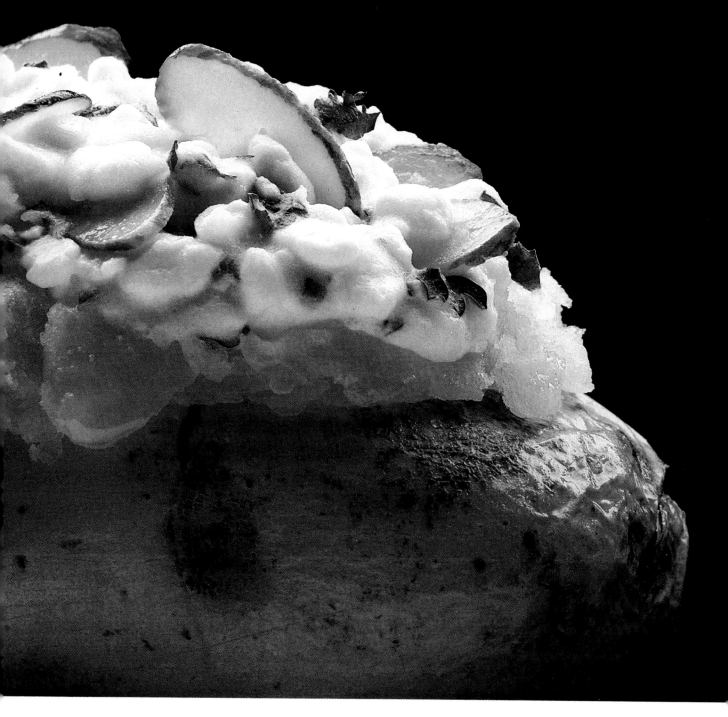

Zesty Stuffed Potatoes ▲

  4 medium baking potatoes
      (8 to 10 oz. each)
 ½ cup cottage cheese
 ¼ cup butter or margarine
 ¼ cup grated Parmesan cheese
 ¼ cup milk
  2 teaspoons prepared
      horseradish
  2 teaspoons dried parsley
      flakes
 ½ cup sliced almonds (optional)

4 servings

Pierce potatoes with fork. Arrange in circle on paper towel in microwave oven. Microwave at High for 10 to 16 minutes, or just until tender, turning over and rearranging once. Let stand for 5 minutes. Cut a thin slice from top of each potato. Scoop out pulp, leaving about ¼-inch shell. Set shells aside.

Place pulp in medium mixing bowl. Add remaining ingredients, except almonds. Beat at medium speed of an electric mixer until blended. Gently stir in almonds. Spoon mixture evenly into potato shells. Arrange potatoes on platter. Microwave at High for 5 to 10 minutes, or until hot, rotating platter once.

Vegetable-topped Potatoes

4 medium baking potatoes (8 to 10 oz. each)
1 pkg. (.87 oz.) white sauce mix
1 cup milk
¼ cup grated Parmesan cheese
¼ teaspoon garlic salt
1 pkg. (10 oz.) frozen chopped broccoli
1 can (8 oz.) corn, drained
½ cup seeded chopped tomato
½ cup shredded Cheddar cheese

4 servings

Pierce potatoes with fork. Arrange in circle on paper towel in micro-wave oven. Microwave at High for 10 to 16 minutes, or just until tender, turning over and rearranging once. Set aside.

In 4-cup measure, blend white sauce mix and milk. Microwave at High for 2½ to 5 minutes, or until sauce thickens and bubbles, stirring 2 or 3 times. Add Parmesan cheese and garlic salt. Mix well. Set aside.

Unwrap broccoli and place on plate. Microwave at High for 4 to 6 min-utes, or until defrosted, turning over and breaking apart once. Drain, pressing to remove excess moisture. In medium bowl, combine broc-coli, corn and tomato. Pour white sauce over vegetables. Toss to coat.

Arrange potatoes on serving plate. Slash each potato lengthwise and then crosswise. Gently press both ends until center pops open. Top each potato with one-fourth of vegetable mixture. Sprinkle evenly with Cheddar cheese. Microwave at 50% (Medium) for 2 to 4 minutes, or until potatoes are hot and cheese is melted, rotating plate once.

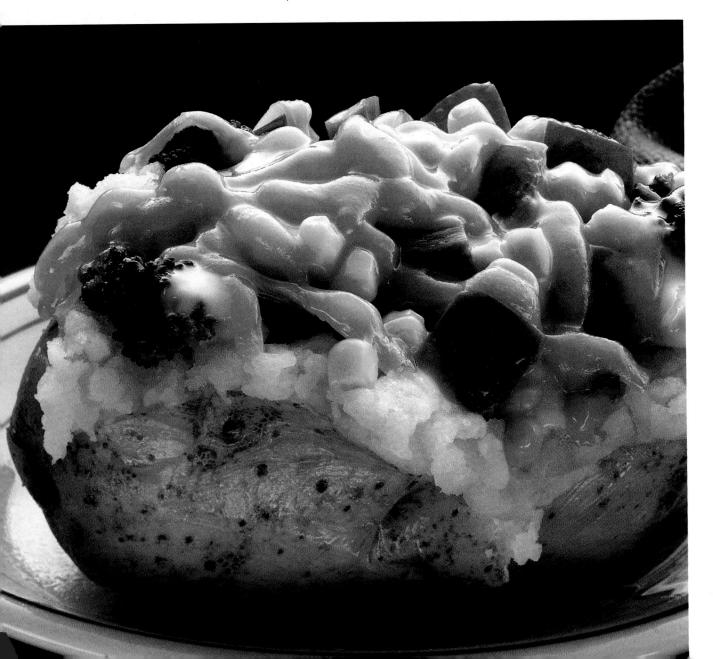

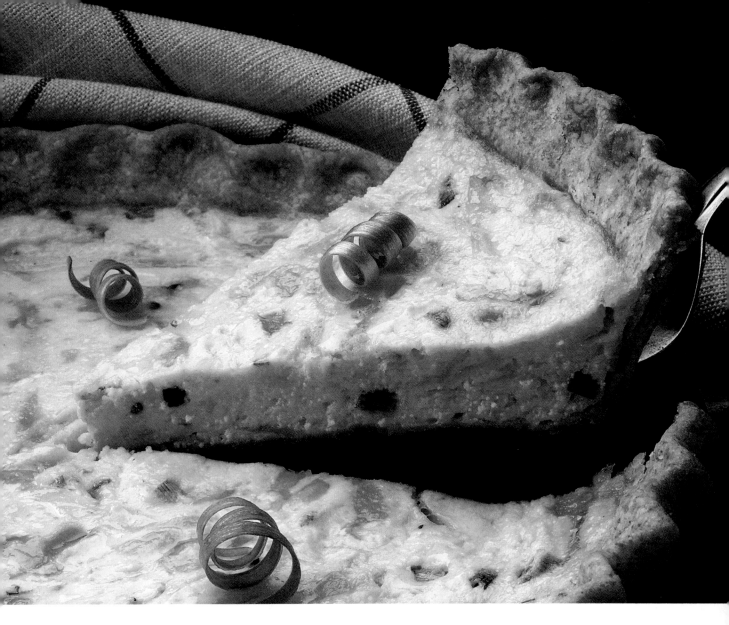

4-Cheese Pie with Whole Wheat Crust

⅔ cup plus 1 tablespoon all-purpose flour, divided
⅓ cup whole wheat flour
½ teaspoon salt
⅓ cup shortening
2 to 3 tablespoons ice water
1 carton (15 oz.) ricotta cheese
3 eggs, beaten
⅓ cup sliced green onions
⅓ cup grated Parmesan cheese
¼ cup evaporated milk
½ teaspoon dried marjoram leaves
½ teaspoon salt
¼ teaspoon pepper
¾ cup shredded Cheddar cheese
½ cup shredded Swiss cheese

4 to 6 servings

In small mixing bowl, combine ⅔ cup all-purpose flour, the wheat flour and salt. Cut in shortening to form coarse crumbs. Sprinkle with water, 1 tablespoon at a time, mixing with fork until particles are moistened and cling together. Form dough into a ball. On lightly floured board, roll out dough at least 2 inches larger than inverted 9-inch pie plate. Ease dough into pie plate. Trim and flute edge. Prick thoroughly. Microwave at High for 5 to 8 minutes, or until crust appears dry and opaque, rotating once or twice. Set aside.

In medium mixing bowl, blend ricotta cheese, remaining 1 tablespoon flour and the eggs. Add remaining ingredients, except Cheddar and Swiss cheeses. Mix well. Stir in cheeses. Pour into prepared crust. Microwave at 70% (Medium High) for 13 to 23 minutes, or until center of filling is set, rotating pie plate 2 or 3 times. Let stand for 10 minutes.

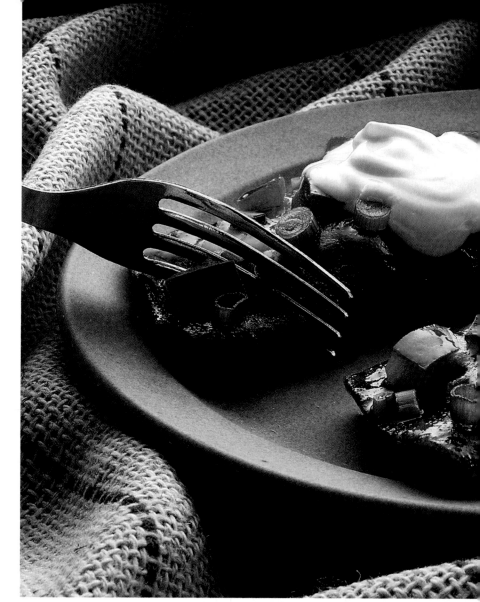

Cheesy Chili Enchiladas ▶

- 1 cup shredded Monterey Jack cheese
- 1 cup shredded Cheddar cheese
- ¼ teaspoon chili powder
- ¼ teaspoon ground cumin
  Vegetable oil
- 6 corn tortillas (6-inch)
- 1 can (10 oz.) enchilada sauce
- 1 can (7 oz.) whole green chilies, drained
  Seeded chopped tomato
  Sliced green onion
  Sour cream

4 to 6 servings

How to Microwave Cheesy Chili Enchiladas

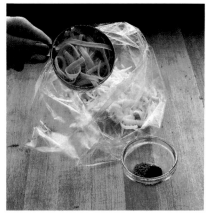

Combine cheeses, chili powder and cumin in large plastic food-storage bag. Shake to coat. Remove ½ cup cheese mixture for topping. Set aside.

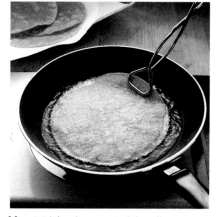

Heat ⅛ inch vegetable oil conventionally in 8-inch skillet over medium-high heat. Dip both sides of each tortilla in hot oil. Place tortillas on paper-towel-lined plate. Set aside.

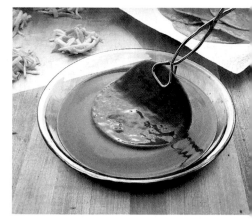

Pour enchilada sauce into shallow dish. Divide remaining cheese mixture into 6 equal portions. To assemble enchiladas, dip both sides of a tortilla in enchilada sauce. Sprinkle 1 portion cheese down the center of tortilla.

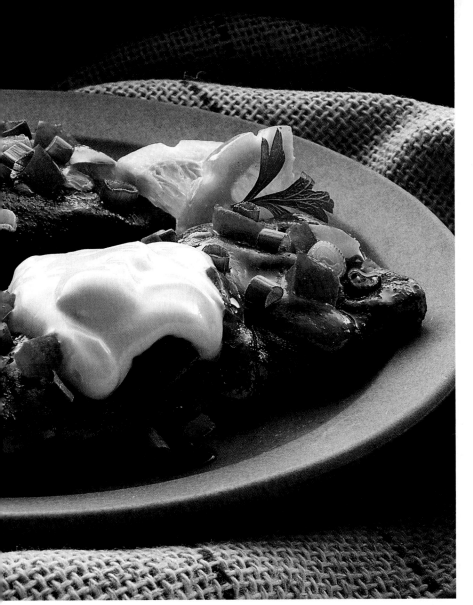

3-Bean Chili

½ cup chopped onion
½ cup chopped celery
⅓ cup chopped green pepper
1 tablespoon olive oil
1 can (28 oz.) whole tomatoes,
    cut up
1 can (15 oz.) tomato sauce
1 can (16 oz.) Great Northern
    beans, rinsed and drained
1 can (15½ oz.) kidney beans,
    rinsed and drained
1 can (15 oz.) garbanzo beans,
    rinsed and drained
2 teaspoons chili powder
1 teaspoon ground cumin
1 teaspoon sugar
½ teaspoon salt
¼ teaspoon garlic powder
⅛ teaspoon pepper
⅛ teaspoon cayenne

8 cups

In 3-quart casserole, combine onion, celery, green pepper and oil. Cover. Microwave at High for 5 to 8 minutes, or until vegetables are tender, stirring once or twice. Add remaining ingredients. Mix well. Re-cover. Microwave at High for 20 to 25 minutes, or until mixture is hot and flavors are blended, stirring 2 or 3 times.

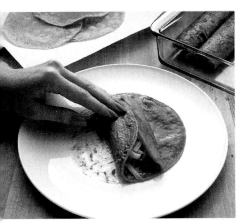

Place 1 green chili in center of tortilla. Roll up tortilla to enclose cheese and chili. Place in 9-inch square baking dish. Repeat with remaining tortillas.

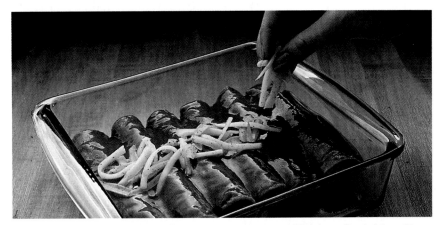

Pour any remaining enchilada sauce over enchiladas. Sprinkle with reserved cheese mixture. Cover with plastic wrap. Microwave at 70% (Medium High) for 8 to 10 minutes, or until enchiladas are hot and cheese is melted, rotating dish 2 or 3 times. Sprinkle with chopped tomato and onion slices. Top with sour cream before serving.

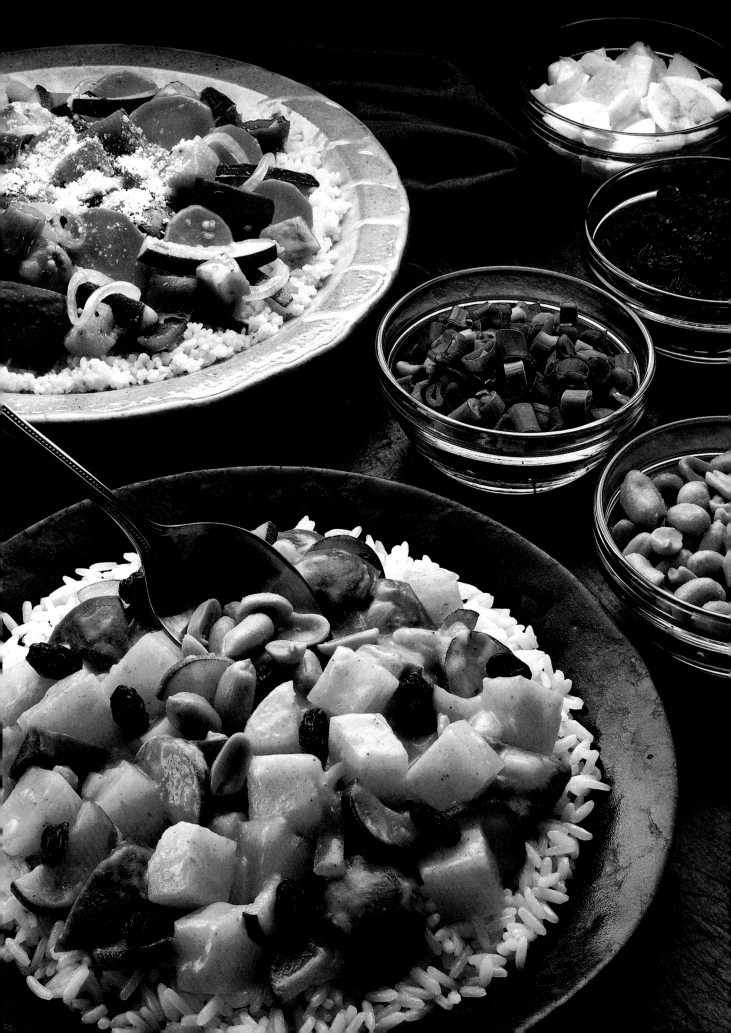

◄ Mediterranean Vegetable Sauté

1 medium green pepper, cut
  into ¾-inch chunks
1 medium onion, thinly sliced
1 cup thinly sliced carrot
2 cloves garlic, minced
⅓ cup olive oil
¾ teaspoon dried marjoram
  leaves
½ teaspoon dried oregano
  leaves

1 small eggplant (about 1 lb.),
  cubed (½-inch cubes)
2 medium zucchini, cut into
  julienne strips (2 × ¼-inch)
1 medium tomato, seeded and
  cut into chunks
¾ teaspoon salt
  Hot cooked couscous
  Grated Parmesan cheese

6 servings

In 3-quart casserole, combine green pepper, onion, carrot, garlic, oil, marjoram and oregano. Mix well. Cover. Microwave at High for 2 to 3½ minutes, or until very hot. Add eggplant and zucchini. Mix well. Re-cover. Microwave at High for 13 to 20 minutes, or until eggplant is tender, stirring 2 or 3 times. Add tomato and salt. Mix well. Re-cover. Let stand for 5 to 10 minutes. Serve over couscous. Top with Parmesan cheese.

◄ Curried Potato & Garden Vegetable Sauce

2 cups cubed potatoes (½-inch
  cubes)
1 small onion, chopped
2 tablespoons butter or
  margarine
1 medium tomato, seeded and
  chopped
1 small zucchini, cut in half
  lengthwise and thinly sliced
1 can (10¾ oz.) condensed
  cream of potato soup

¾ cup milk
1 to 1½ teaspoons curry
  powder
¼ teaspoon salt
  Hot cooked rice

Condiments:
  Raisins
  Chopped hard-cooked eggs
  Chopped peanuts
  Sliced green onions

4 to 6 servings

In 2-quart casserole, combine potatoes, chopped onion and butter. Cover. Microwave at High for 7 to 10 minutes, or until potatoes are tender, stirring once or twice. Add remaining ingredients, except rice and condiments. Mix well. Re-cover. Microwave at High for 7 to 9 minutes, or until sauce is hot and flavors are blended, stirring once or twice. Serve over rice. Sprinkle each serving with desired condiments.

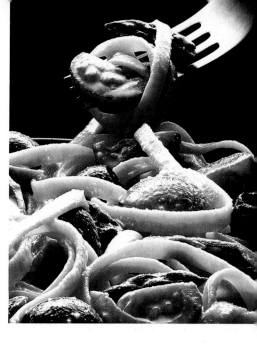

Fresh Vegetable Alfredo ▲

½ lb. fresh asparagus, cut into
  ¾-inch lengths
¼ cup butter or margarine
1 can (16 oz.) pitted black olives
½ cup whipping cream
2 eggs, beaten
½ cup grated Parmesan cheese
⅛ teaspoon garlic powder
⅛ teaspoon pepper
8 oz. uncooked fettuccini
1 cup quartered cherry
  tomatoes

4 servings

In 2-quart casserole, place asparagus and butter. Cover. Microwave at High for 3 to 4 minutes, or until butter is melted and asparagus is tender-crisp, stirring once. Add olives. Set aside. In small mixing bowl, blend whipping cream, eggs, Parmesan cheese, garlic powder and pepper. Add to asparagus mixture. Mix well. Set aside.

Prepare fettuccini as directed on package. Rinse and drain. Add to asparagus mixture. Toss to coat. Microwave at 50% (Medium) for 4 to 6 minutes, or until hot, stirring every 2 minutes. Add cherry tomatoes. Toss to combine. Before serving, sprinkle with additional grated Parmesan cheese if desired.

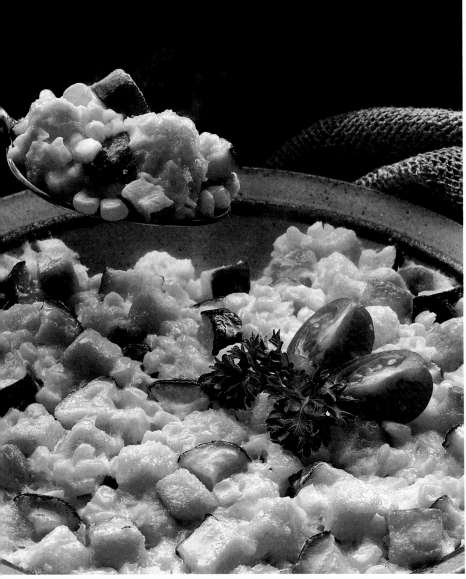

◄ Scalloped Vegetable Bake

1½ cups cubed zucchini
    (½-inch cubes)
 1 cup frozen corn
¼ cup chopped onion
 2 tablespoons butter or
    margarine
 1 tablespoon all-purpose flour
½ teaspoon salt
 2 cups onion and garlic-
    seasoned croutons
1½ cups shredded Swiss cheese
 1 cup milk
 2 eggs, beaten

4 servings

In 1½-quart casserole, combine zucchini, corn, onion and butter. Cover. Microwave at High for 5 to 9 minutes, or until vegetables are tender-crisp, stirring once. Add flour and salt. Mix well. Stir in croutons and cheese.

In 2-cup measure, blend milk and eggs. Pour over vegetable mixture. Let stand for 15 minutes. Microwave at High for 17½ to 22½ minutes, or until mixture is set, rotating 3 times. Let stand for 5 minutes. Before serving, garnish with fresh parsley sprigs and cherry tomatoes, if desired.

Crunchy Wild Rice Casserole

 1 cup uncooked wild rice
 2 tablespoons butter or
    margarine
⅓ cup chopped pecans
 1 cup sliced fresh mushrooms
⅓ cup chopped celery
½ teaspoon dried marjoram
    leaves
½ teaspoon salt
⅛ teaspoon pepper
 3 tablespoons all-purpose flour
 1 can (12 oz.) evaporated
    skimmed milk
 1 cup cubed smoked Cheddar
    cheese (½-inch cubes)

4 servings

Prepare wild rice as directed on package. Drain and set aside. In 2-quart casserole, microwave butter at High for 45 seconds to 1 minute, or until melted. Add pecans. Toss to coat. Microwave at High for 1½ to 2½ minutes, or until hot and bubbly.

Add mushrooms, celery and seasonings. Mix well. Cover. Microwave at High for 2 to 3 minutes, or until vegetables are tender, stirring once or twice. Stir in flour. Blend in evaporated milk. Re-cover. Microwave at High for 8 to 11 minutes, or until mixture is thick and creamy. Stir in cheese cubes. Re-cover. Let stand for 5 minutes.

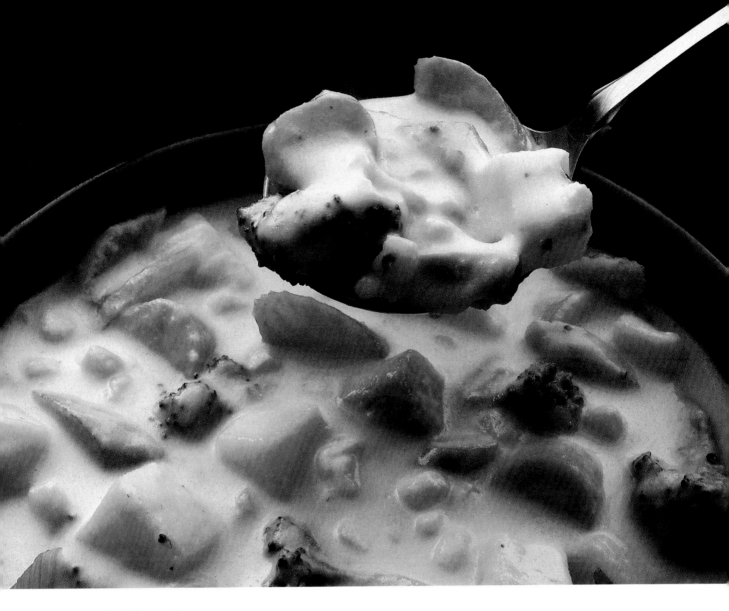

Vegetable Chowder

- 1 pkg. (10 oz.) frozen chopped broccoli
- 1 medium potato, cut into ½-inch cubes
- ½ cup chopped carrot
- ⅓ cup chopped celery
- ½ teaspoon dried marjoram leaves
- 3 tablespoons butter or margarine
- 3 tablespoons all-purpose flour
- ½ teaspoon salt
- 1⅔ cups milk
- 1½ cups shredded Cheddar cheese
- ½ cup frozen corn
  Cheddar cheese croutons (optional)

6 to 8 servings

Unwrap broccoli and place on plate. Microwave at High for 4 to 6 minutes, or until defrosted, turning over and breaking apart once. Drain. Set aside.

In 2-quart casserole, combine potato, carrot, celery, marjoram and butter. Cover. Microwave at High for 6 to 11 minutes, or until vegetables are tender, stirring once. Stir in flour and salt. Blend in milk. Microwave, uncovered, at High for 6½ to 9 minutes, or until chowder thickens and bubbles, stirring once or twice. Add cheese. Stir until cheese melts.

Add broccoli and corn to chowder. Stir. Cover. Microwave at High for 3 to 8 minutes, or until hot, stirring once. Top with croutons.

Italian Eggplant Bake

⅓ cup olive oil
1 large clove garlic, minced
¾ teaspoon dried basil leaves, divided
½ teaspoon dried oregano leaves, divided
8 eggplant slices (½ inch thick), peeled
2 cups shredded mozzarella or Provolone cheese
1 can (15 oz.) tomato purée
¼ teaspoon salt

4 servings

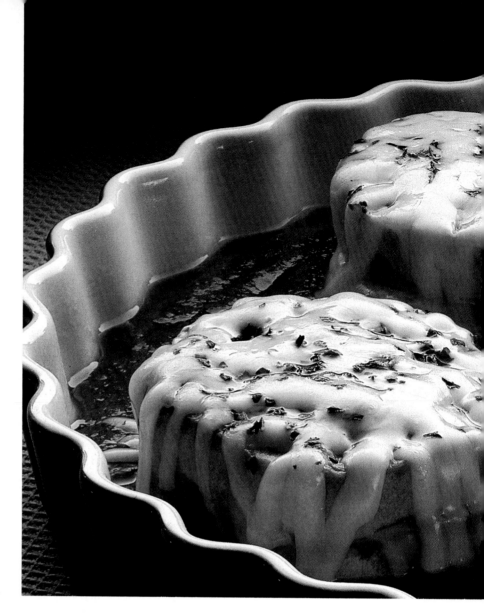

How to Microwave Italian Eggplant Bake

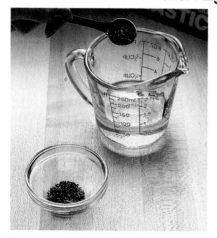

Combine oil, garlic, ½ teaspoon basil and ¼ teaspoon oregano in 1-cup measure. Cover with plastic wrap. Microwave at High for 45 seconds to 1 minute, or just until warm. Let stand for 5 minutes.

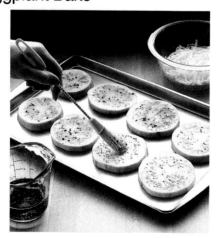

Brush both sides of each eggplant slice with oil mixture. Arrange slices in single layer on baking sheet. Add remaining oil mixture to cheese. Toss to coat. Set aside.

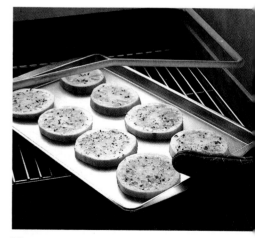

Place eggplant slices under conventional broiler, 3 to 4 inches from heat. Broil until lightly browned, 4 to 6 minutes. Turn slices over and broil until lightly browned, 4 to 6 minutes longer.

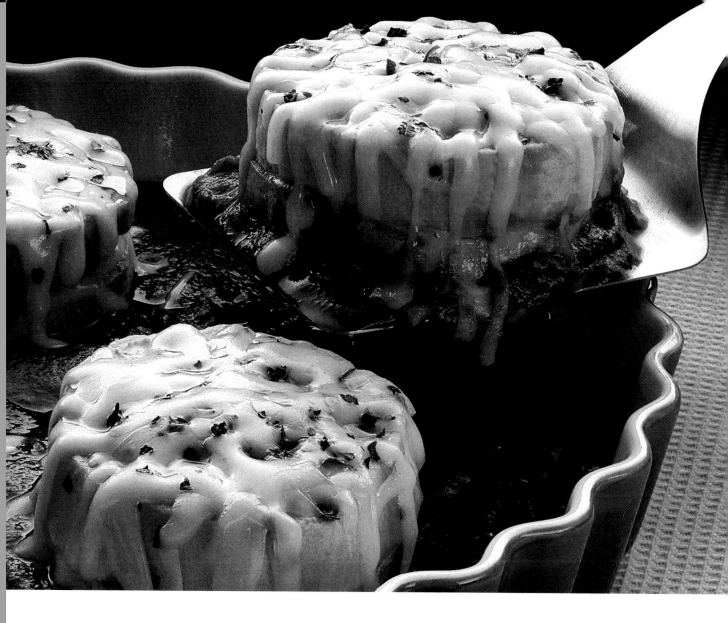

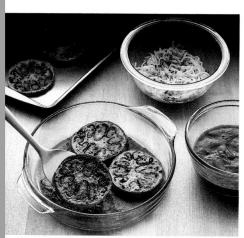

Combine tomato purée, salt, remaining ¼ teaspoon basil and oregano in small bowl. Spread ¼ cup tomato mixture in bottom of 9-inch round baking dish. Arrange 4 eggplant slices on top of tomato mixture.

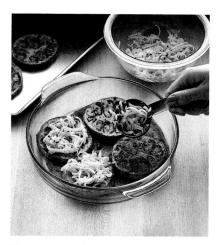

Top each slice with a scant ¼ cup cheese mixture. Top with remaining eggplant slices and cheese.

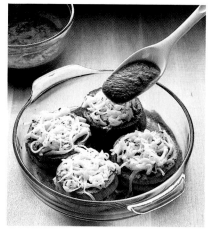

Spoon remaining purée around eggplant. Cover with plastic wrap. Microwave at 70% (Medium High) for 7½ to 10 minutes, or until hot and bubbly around edges, rotating dish 2 or 3 times.

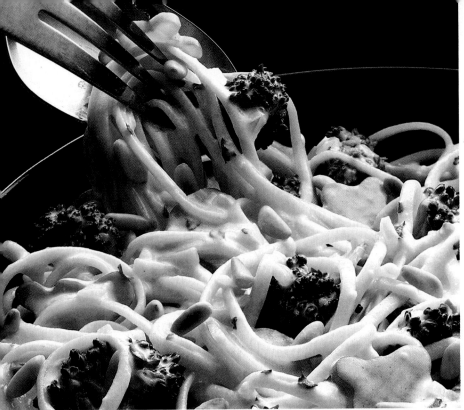

Linguine & Red-Peppered Broccoli

- ¼ cup pine nuts
- 8 oz. uncooked linguine
- 1 medium head broccoli
  (1 to 1½ lbs.)
- ½ teaspoon crushed red
  pepper flakes
- 2 tablespoons olive oil
- 3 tablespoons water
- ½ cup chopped onion
- 3 tablespoons butter or
  margarine, cut up
- 1 clove garlic, minced
- 3 tablespoons all-purpose flour
- 1 teaspoon dried parsley flakes
- ¾ teaspoon salt
- 2 cups half-and-half
- 4 to 6 drops red pepper sauce
  (optional)

4 to 6 servings

Place pine nuts in small skillet. Cook conventionally over medium heat just until golden, stirring constantly. Place in small bowl and set aside. Prepare linguine as directed on package. Rinse and drain. Set aside.

Cut broccoli into small flowerets, and thinly slice stalks. Place in 3-quart casserole. Add red pepper flakes and olive oil. Toss to coat. Sprinkle with water. Cover. Microwave at High for 6 to 8 minutes, or until tender-crisp, stirring once. Drain. Add linguine. Mix well. Set aside.

In 2-quart casserole, combine onion, butter and garlic. Cover. Microwave at High for 2½ to 4 minutes, or until butter is melted and onion is tender. Stir in flour, parsley and salt. Blend in half-and-half and red pepper sauce. Microwave at High for 6½ to 11 minutes or until mixture thickens and bubbles, stirring 2 or 3 times. Pour over broccoli mixture. Toss to coat. Sprinkle with pine nuts.

Florentine Mostaccioli Bake

- 1 pkg. (10 oz.) frozen
  chopped spinach
- 3 tablespoons butter or
  margarine
- ⅓ cup chopped onion
- 3 tablespoons all-purpose
  flour
- ¼ teaspoon salt
- ⅛ teaspoon ground nutmeg
- ⅛ teaspoon pepper
- 1½ cups half-and-half
- ½ cup grated Parmesan
  cheese
- 8 oz. uncooked mostaccioli

Topping:
- 2 tablespoons butter or
  margarine
- ½ cup seasoned dry bread
  crumbs
- 1 tablespoon grated
  Parmesan cheese

4 servings

Unwrap spinach and place on plate. Microwave at High for 4 to 6 minutes, or until defrosted, turning over and breaking apart once. Drain, pressing to remove excess moisture. Set aside.

In 2-quart casserole, combine 3 tablespoons butter and the onion. Cover. Microwave at High for 3 to 4½ minutes, or until butter is melted and onion is tender, stirring once. Stir in flour, salt, nutmeg and pepper. Blend in half-and-half. Microwave at High for 5 to 6 minutes, or until mixture thickens and bubbles, stirring 2 or 3 times. Add spinach and ½ cup Parmesan cheese. Mix well.

Prepare mostaccioli as directed on package. Rinse and drain. Add to sauce. Mix well. Cover. Microwave at High for 4 to 7½ minutes, or until hot, stirring once or twice. Set aside.

In small mixing bowl, microwave 2 tablespoons butter at High for 45 seconds to 1 minute, or until melted. Add remaining topping ingredients. Mix well. Sprinkle over casserole. Microwave at High for 2 to 3 minutes, or until topping is hot. Before serving, garnish casserole with snipped fresh parsley and whole black olives, if desired.

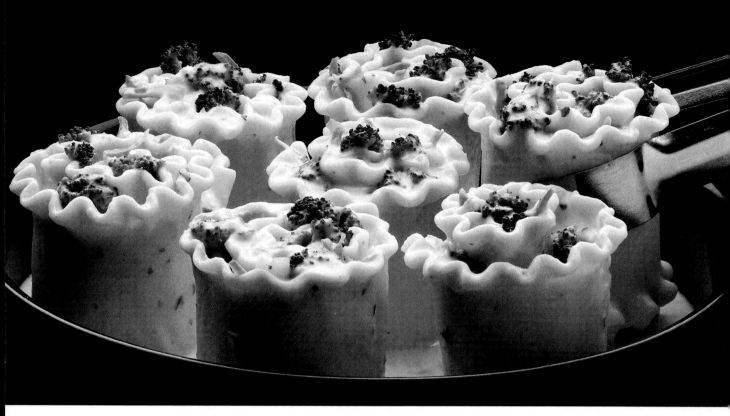

Vegetable Lasagna Spirals

8 uncooked spinach or egg
    lasagna noodles

Vegetable Mixture:
1 pkg. (10 oz.) frozen chopped
    broccoli
½ cup shredded carrot
¼ cup chopped onion
2 tablespoons butter or
    margarine
¼ teaspoon dried thyme leaves

Cheese Filling:
1 carton (15 oz.) ricotta cheese
¼ cup grated Parmesan cheese
1 egg, beaten
¼ teaspoon dried thyme leaves
⅛ teaspoon garlic powder

Sauce:
1 package (.87 oz.) white
    sauce mix
1 cup milk
1 teaspoon dried parsley flakes
1 cup shredded Monterey Jack
    cheese

4 to 6 servings

Prepare lasagna noodles as directed on package. Drain. Cover with cool water. Set aside. In 2-quart casserole, combine all vegetable mixture ingredients. Cover. Microwave at High for 7½ to 12 minutes, or until vegetables are tender, stirring 2 or 3 times. Set aside. In medium mixing bowl, combine all cheese filling ingredients. Mix well. Set aside.

In 4-cup measure, blend white sauce mix, milk and parsley. Microwave at High for 2½ to 5 minutes, or until mixture thickens and bubbles, stirring 2 or 3 times. Stir in cheese. Set aside.

Remove lasagna noodles from water and place on damp paper towels. To assemble spirals, spread about ¼ cup cheese mixture onto each noodle. Sprinkle with about ¼ cup vegetable mixture. Roll up noodle to enclose filling. Arrange spirals on end in 9-inch round baking dish. Pour sauce evenly around spirals. Cover with plastic wrap. Microwave at 50% (Medium) for 14 to 20 minutes, or until spirals are hot, rotating dish 2 or 3 times.

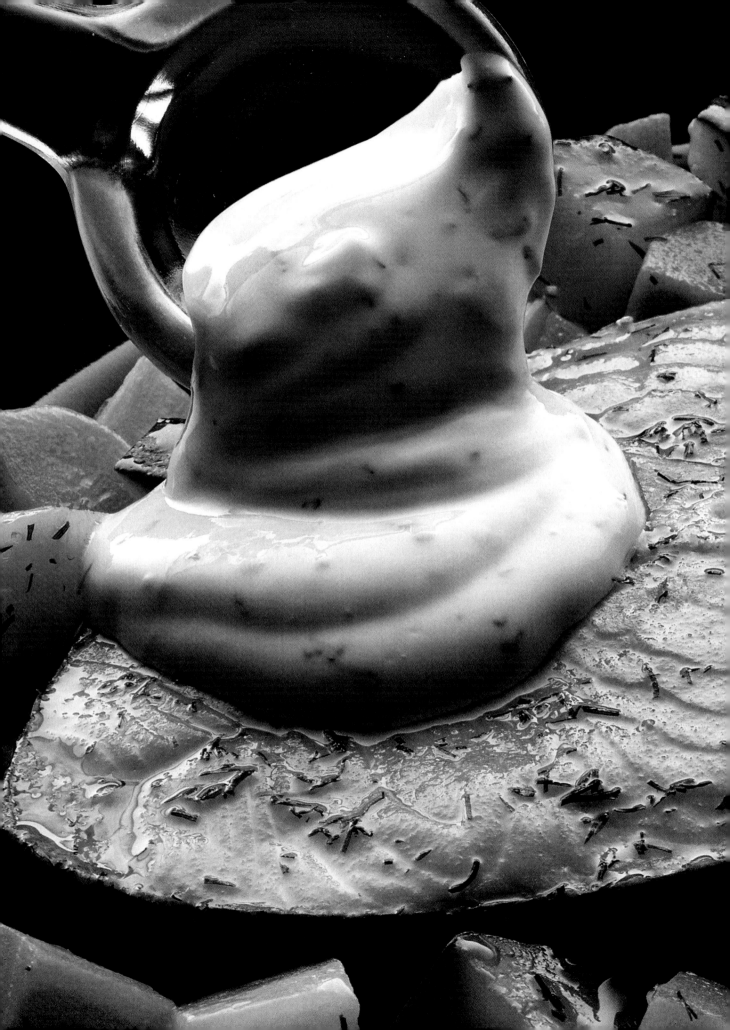

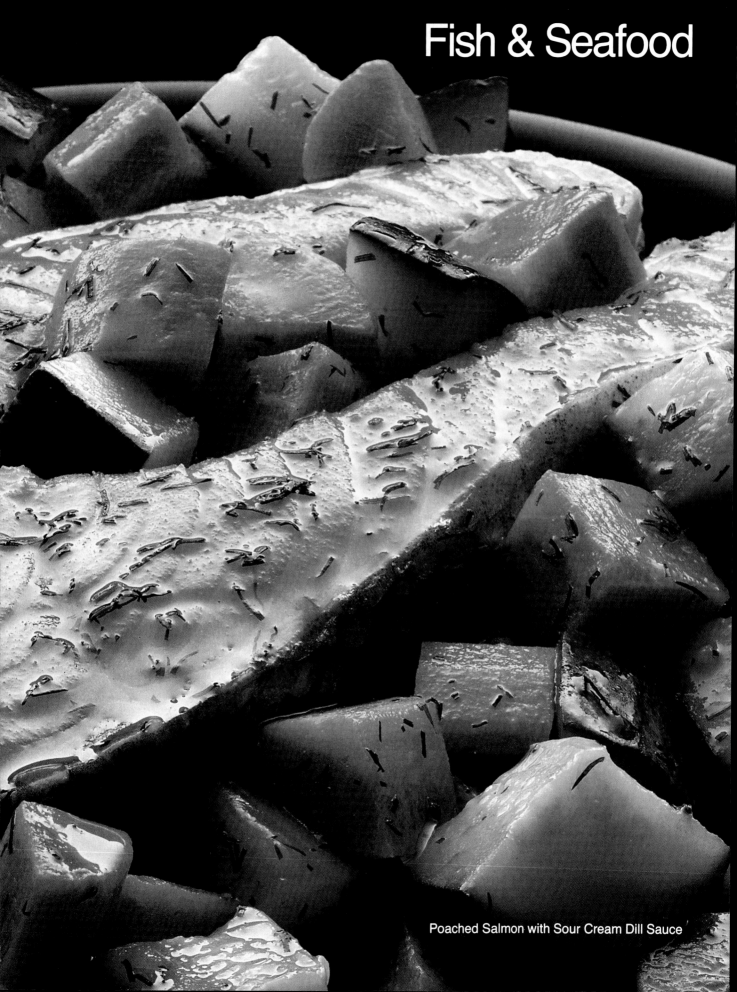

Poached Salmon with Sour Cream Dill Sauce

Neptune Torte

Crepes:

- 1 tablespoon butter or margarine
- 1¼ cups milk
- 1 cup all-purpose flour
- 1 egg
- ¼ teaspoon salt

Filling:

- 2 tablespoons butter or margarine
- 2 tablespoons all-purpose flour
- 1 teaspoon dried basil leaves
- ¾ cup milk
- 2 tablespoons white wine
- 1 cup shredded Monterey Jack cheese
- 1 can (6 oz.) crab meat, rinsed, drained and cartilage removed
- 1 can (4¼ oz.) small shrimp, rinsed and drained
- 1 tablespoon sliced green onion

4 servings

How to Microwave a Neptune Torte

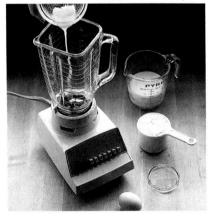

Place 1 tablespoon butter in small bowl. Microwave at High for 45 seconds to 1 minute, or until melted. In blender or food processor, place melted butter and remaining crepe ingredients. Process until mixture is smooth. Chill for at least 1 hour.

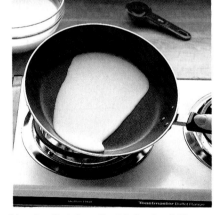

Heat a lightly oiled 6-inch skillet conventionally over medium heat. Pour about 3 tablespoons crepe batter into skillet. Tilt skillet in a circular motion to coat bottom with a thin layer of batter.

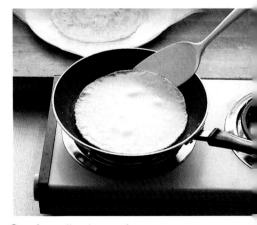

Cook until edges of crepe are set and begin to pull away from edges of pan. Turn and brown other side. Repeat to yield 6 crepes. Stack crepes between wax paper and set aside. Any additional crepes may be frozen for later use.

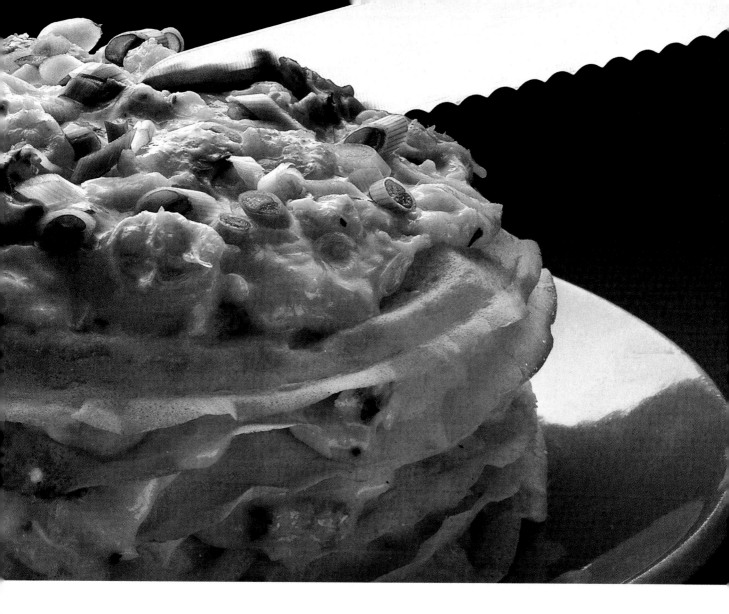

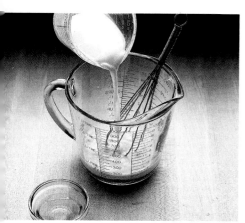

Place 2 tablespoons butter in 4-cup measure. Microwave at High for 45 seconds to 1 minute, or until melted. Stir in flour and basil. Blend in milk and wine. Microwave at High for 3 to 4 minutes, or until mixture thickens and bubbles, stirring 2 or 3 times. Stir in cheese, crab meat and shrimp.

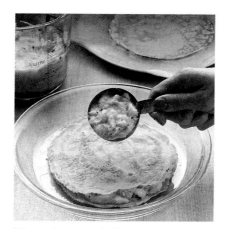

Place 1 crepe in bottom of 9-inch pie plate. Top with ⅓ cup seafood mixture. Spread to within ½ inch of edge. Repeat layers, ending with seafood mixture.

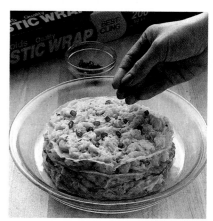

Sprinkle top with green onion. Cover with plastic wrap. Microwave at 50% (Medium) for 7 to 9 minutes, or until hot and bubbly around edges, rotating dish 2 or 3 times. Serve torte in wedges.

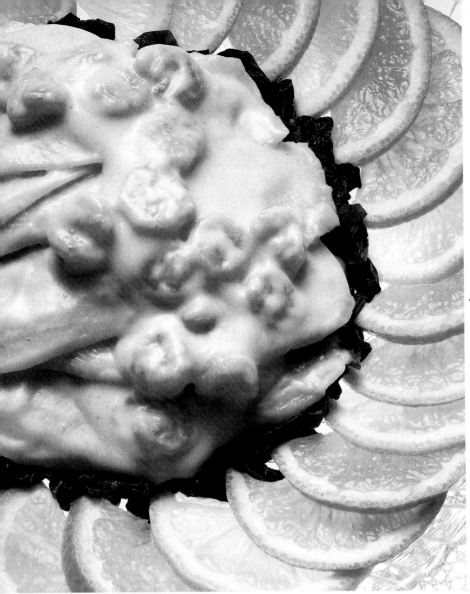

Citrus-sauced Shrimp & Fillets

- 1 tablespoon butter or margarine
- ¼ teaspoon grated lemon peel
- ¼ teaspoon grated orange peel
- 1 tablespoon all-purpose flour
- ¼ teaspoon salt
- ⅛ teaspoon ground nutmeg
- ½ cup milk
- 1 pkg. (10 oz.) frozen sole fillets
- 1 can (4¼ oz.) small shrimp, rinsed and drained
- 1 pkg. (10 oz.) frozen chopped spinach
- 2 tablespoons water

4 servings

In 9-inch square baking dish, place butter and lemon and orange peels. Cover with plastic wrap. Microwave at High for 45 seconds to 1 minute, or until butter melts. Stir in flour, salt and nutmeg. Blend in milk. Arrange frozen fish fillets in a single layer in dish. Cover with plastic wrap. Microwave at 70% (Medium High) for 12 to 16 minutes, or until fish flakes easily with fork, stirring sauce 2 or 3 times. Stir in shrimp. Set aside.

In 1-quart casserole, place spinach and water. Cover. Microwave at High for 4 to 6 minutes, or until spinach is hot, stirring once to break apart. Drain. Arrange spinach on serving platter in an even layer. Top with fillets. Spoon sauce over fillets. Garnish with orange and lemon slices, if desired.

Lemon-Dijon Fillets

- ¾ lb. fish fillets, about ½ inch thick, cut into serving-size pieces
  Lemon pepper seasoning (optional)
- 1 tablespoon plus 1 teaspoon butter or margarine
- 1 tablespoon plus 1 teaspoon all-purpose flour
- 1 teaspoon grated lemon peel
- ½ teaspoon dried parsley flakes
- ⅛ teaspoon salt
- ⅔ cup milk
- 1 to 2 teaspoons Dijon mustard
- ⅔ cup seeded finely chopped tomato (optional)

4 servings

In 9-inch square baking dish, arrange fish with thickest portions toward outside of dish. Sprinkle lightly with lemon pepper. Cover with plastic wrap. Microwave at High for 3½ to 5½ minutes, or until fish flakes easily with fork, rotating dish once. Set aside, covered.

In small bowl, microwave butter at High for 45 seconds to 1 minute, or until melted. Stir in flour, lemon peel, parsley and salt. Blend in milk. Microwave at High for 1½ to 3 minutes, or until mixture thickens and bubbles, stirring once or twice. Add mustard. Mix well. Arrange fish on serving platter. Top with sauce. Garnish with chopped tomato.

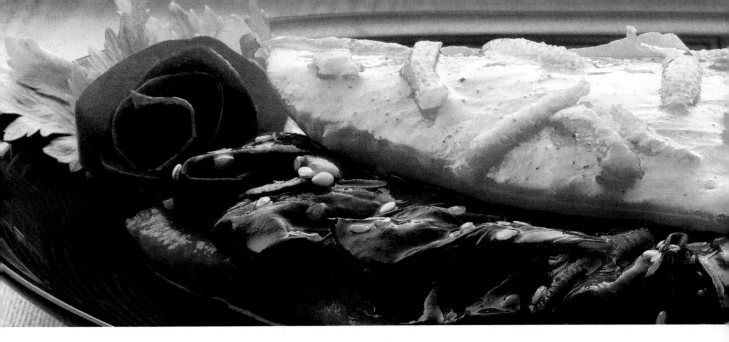

Fillets Florentine ▲ with Sesame Butter

¼ lb. fresh spinach, trimmed and torn, about 2 cups
1 teaspoon sesame seed
1 teaspoon sesame oil, divided
¼ cup butter or margarine
⅛ teaspoon cayenne
8 fish fillets (2 oz. each), about ¼ inch thick*
1 to 2 teaspoons grated orange peel

4 servings

In medium mixing bowl, combine spinach, sesame seed and ½ teaspoon sesame oil. Toss to coat. Set aside. In small bowl, combine butter, remaining ½ teaspoon sesame oil and the cayenne. Microwave at High for 1¼ to 1½ minutes, or until butter melts. Set aside.

Place 4 fish fillets on roasting rack. Brush with butter mixture. Top each fillet with one-fourth of spinach mixture. Top with remaining fillets. Brush with butter mixture. Sprinkle evenly with grated orange peel. Microwave at 70% (Medium High) for 7½ to 12½ minutes, or until fish flakes easily with fork, rotating rack once or twice. Drizzle fillets with any remaining butter mixture.

*Fillets should be of equal size and shape.

Mushroom-topped Fillets

8 oz. fresh mushrooms, finely chopped
½ cup chopped onion
2 tablespoons butter or margarine
1 teaspoon dried parsley flakes
¾ lb. fish fillets, about ½ inch thick, cut into serving-size pieces
1 tablespoon chopped pimiento
¼ teaspoon salt
Sour cream (optional)

4 servings

In 1½-quart casserole, combine mushrooms, onion, butter and parsley. Microwave, uncovered, at High for 5 to 7 minutes, or until onion is tender, stirring once. Cover. Set aside.

In 9-inch square baking dish, arrange fish fillets with thickest portions toward outside of dish. Cover with plastic wrap. Microwave at High for 3½ to 5½ minutes, or until fish flakes easily with fork, rotating dish once. Re-cover. Set aside. If necessary, microwave mushroom mixture at High for 1 to 2 minutes, or until hot. Drain. Stir in pimiento and salt. Arrange fish on serving platter. Top with mushroom mixture. Garnish with sour cream.

Mexican Salsa Fillets

2 medium tomatoes, seeded and chopped
½ cup chopped onion
2 tablespoons chopped green chilies
2 teaspoons olive oil
1 clove garlic, minced
¼ teaspoon ground cumin
¼ teaspoon salt
⅛ teaspoon dried oregano leaves
Dash crushed red pepper flakes
¾ lb. fish fillets, about ½ inch thick, cut into serving-size pieces

4 servings

In 1½-quart casserole, combine all ingredients, except fish fillets. Mix well. Microwave, uncovered, at High for 20 to 28 minutes, or until salsa is desired consistency, stirring once. Set aside.

In 9-inch square baking dish, arrange fish fillets with thickest portions toward outside of dish. Cover with plastic wrap. Microwave at High for 3½ to 5½ minutes, or until fish flakes easily with fork, rotating dish once. Let stand, covered, for 3 minutes. If necessary, microwave salsa at High for 1 to 2 minutes or until hot. Arrange fish on serving platter. Top with salsa.

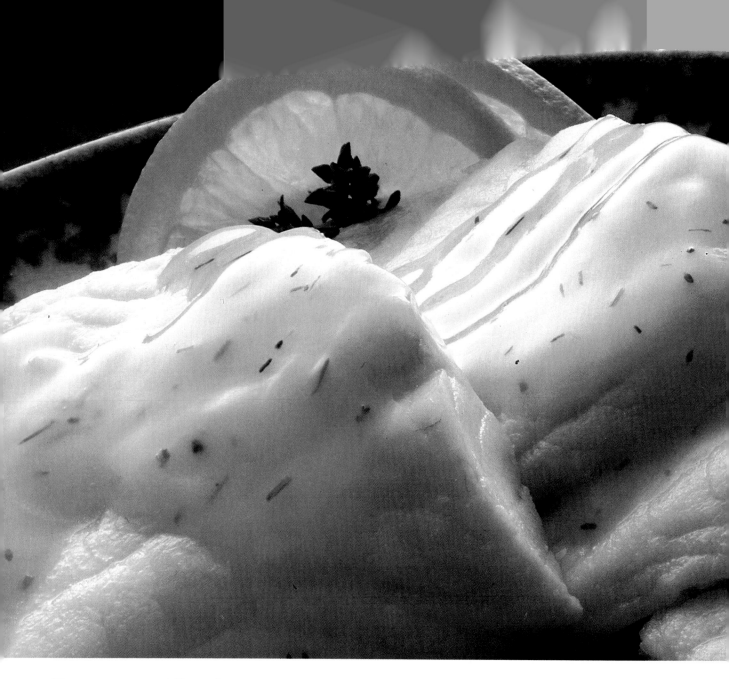

Orange-sauced Roughy ▲

½ cup fresh orange juice
⅓ cup white wine or
   ready-to-serve chicken broth
2 teaspoons cornstarch
1 teaspoon sugar
   Dash dried thyme leaves
¾ lb. orange roughy fillets,
   about ½ inch thick, cut into
   serving-size pieces

4 servings

In 2-cup measure, blend all ingredients, except fish. Microwave at High for 2½ to 4½ minutes, or until sauce is thickened and translucent, stirring once or twice. Set aside.

In 9-inch square baking dish, arrange fish with thickest portions toward outside. Cover with plastic wrap. Microwave at High for 3½ to 5½ minutes, or until fish flakes easily with fork, rotating dish once. Let stand, covered, for 2 minutes. If necessary, microwave sauce at High for 1 minute, or until hot. Arrange fish on serving platter. Top with sauce.

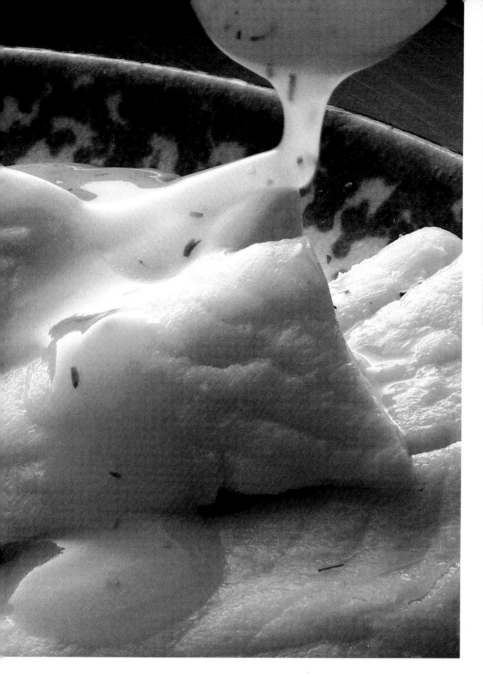

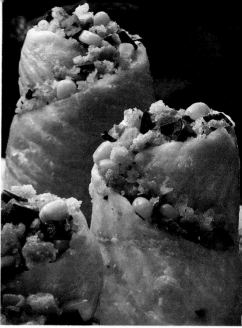

Cajun Stuffed Sole ▲

⅓ cup chopped red or green
   pepper
2 tablespoons sliced green
   onion
2 tablespoons butter or
   margarine
1 teaspoon dried parsley flakes
¼ teaspoon cayenne
¼ teaspoon salt
⅛ teaspoon pepper
1 cup corn bread stuffing mix
1 can (8 oz.) corn, drained
2 tablespoons ready-to-serve
   chicken broth or water
4 sole fillets (8 oz. each), about
   ¼ inch thick and 10
   inches long

4 servings

In 1-quart casserole, combine red pepper, onion, butter, parsley, cayenne, salt and pepper. Cover. Microwave at High for 2 to 3 minutes, or until vegetables are tender, stirring once. Add remaining ingredients, except sole. Mix well.

Spread one-fourth of stuffing down the center of each fillet. Roll up fillet, enclosing stuffing. Secure with wooden pick. Stand stuffed fillets on end in 9-inch pie plate. Cover with plastic wrap. Microwave at 70% (Medium High) for 8 to 10 minutes, or until center of fish roll flakes easily with fork, rotating dish once or twice. Let stand, covered, for 3 minutes.

Cod & Tomato Bake

1 medium onion, cut into
   wedges
1 tablespoon olive oil
¼ teaspoon dried thyme leaves
1 can (16 oz.) stewed tomatoes
1 pkg. (10 oz.) frozen cod fillets

Topping:
⅓ cup crushed Cheddar cheese
   crackers
1 tablespoon grated Parmesan
   cheese
1 teaspoon dried parsley flakes

4 servings

In 9-inch square baking dish, place onion, oil and thyme. Cover with plastic wrap. Microwave at High for 4 to 8 minutes, or until onion is tender, stirring once. Add tomatoes. Mix well. Arrange frozen cod fillets over tomato mixture. Re-cover. Microwave at High for 8 to 11 minutes, or until fish flakes easily with fork, rotating dish 2 or 3 times.

In small bowl, combine all topping ingredients. Mix well. Spoon mixture evenly over cod pieces. Microwave at High for 1 to 2 minutes, or until hot.

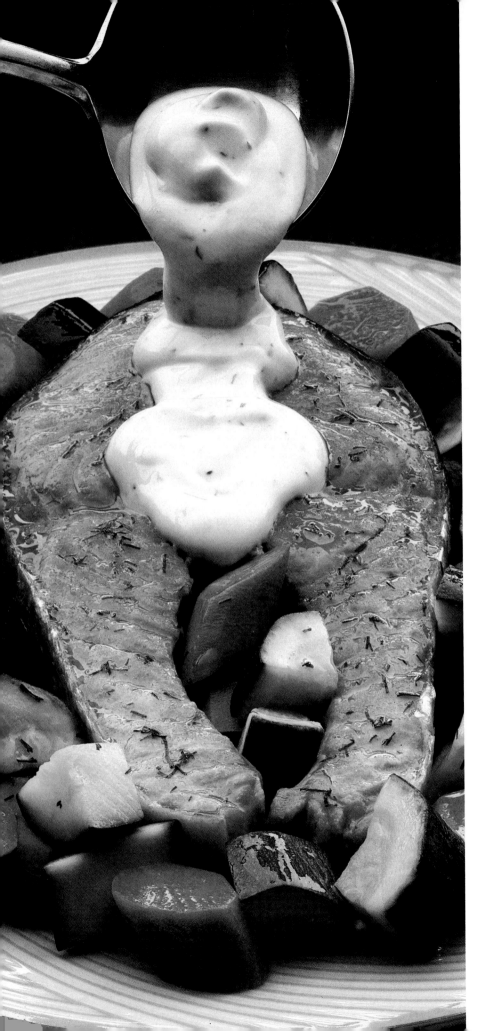

Poached Salmon with Sour Cream Dill Sauce

Sauce:
½ cup sour cream
1 tablespoon milk
¼ teaspoon dried dill weed

Poaching Liquid:
1 can (14½ oz.) ready-to-serve chicken broth
2 medium carrots, cut into ½-inch chunks
½ teaspoon dried dill weed
⅛ teaspoon dried celery seed

4 salmon steaks (8 oz. each), about ¾ inch thick
1 medium zucchini, cut into ½-inch cubes

4 servings

In small bowl, combine all sauce ingredients. Chill for 30 minutes to blend flavors. In 9-inch square baking dish, combine chicken broth, carrots, ½ teaspoon dill weed and the celery seed. Cover with plastic wrap. Microwave at High for 5 to 9 minutes, or until mixture boils.

Arrange salmon steaks in baking dish with meaty portions toward outside edges. Re-cover. Microwave at 70% (Medium High) for 10 to 15 minutes, or until salmon flakes easily with fork, rotating dish 2 or 3 times. Top salmon evenly with zucchini. Re-cover. Microwave at 70% (Medium High) for 2 minutes longer. Let stand, covered, for 5 minutes.

Arrange salmon steaks on a serving plate. Strain poaching liquid from vegetables. Discard liquid. Arrange vegetables around steaks. Serve with sauce.

Halibut Veronique ▶

2 halibut steaks (12 oz. each), about 1 inch thick
1 cup sliced fresh mushrooms
2 tablespoons butter or margarine, cut up
1 tablespoon sliced green onion
½ teaspoon dried tarragon leaves
¼ teaspoon celery salt
1 tablespoon cornstarch
⅔ cup ready-to-serve chicken broth
¼ cup white wine
½ cup seedless green grapes, cut in half

4 servings

Cut bone from center of each halibut steak, using thin blade of knife and being careful not to slice all the way through ends of steak. Cut each steak in half crosswise to yield 4 pieces. Set halibut aside.

In 9-inch square baking dish, combine mushrooms, butter, onion, tarragon and celery salt. Cover dish with plastic wrap. Microwave at High for 3 to 4 minutes, or until vegetables are tender, stirring once. Stir in cornstarch. Blend in chicken broth and wine.

Arrange halibut steaks in baking dish with meaty portions toward outside edges. Spoon broth mixture over steaks. Microwave at 70% (Medium High) for 11 to 14 minutes, or until fish flakes easily with fork, rotating dish and stirring sauce once or twice. Before serving, sprinkle with grapes.

Scandinavian Fish Patties

Topping:
⅓ cup mayonnaise
1 to 2 teaspoons prepared horseradish

Patties:
2 tablespoons chopped celery
2 tablespoons sliced green onion
1 tablespoon butter or margarine
1 cup instant mashed potato flakes

1 can (6½ oz.) water-pack tuna, drained
¾ cup milk
1 teaspoon prepared horseradish
⅛ teaspoon garlic powder
⅛ teaspoon celery seed

Coating:
½ cup cornflake crumbs
1 teaspoon dried parsley flakes
½ teaspoon paprika

4 servings

In small bowl, mix topping ingredients. Chill until serving time. In 1-quart casserole, place celery, onion and butter. Cover. Microwave at High for 1½ to 2½ minutes, or until vegetables are tender, stirring once. Add remaining patty ingredients. Mix well. Set aside. In shallow dish, combine all coating ingredients.

Shape tuna mixture into 4 patties, about ½ inch thick. Dip each patty into crumb mixture, pressing to coat. Arrange patties on roasting rack. Microwave at High for 3½ to 5 minutes, or until hot, rotating rack once. Serve with prepared topping. Sprinkle with sliced green onion, if desired.

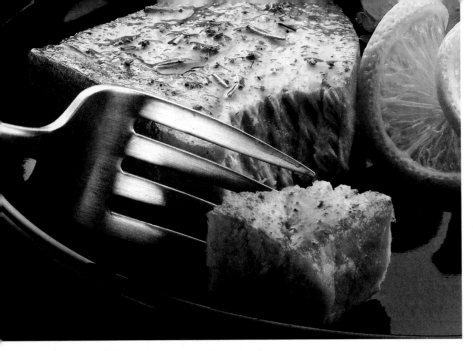

Herb-seasoned Swordfish Steaks ▲

2 tablespoons vegetable oil
¼ teaspoon dried rosemary leaves
¼ teaspoon dried thyme leaves
¼ teaspoon paprika

⅛ teaspoon garlic powder
⅛ teaspoon salt
1 swordfish steak (1½ lbs.), about 1 inch thick, cut into 4 serving-size pieces

4 servings

In small bowl, combine all ingredients, except swordfish. Mix well. Microwave at High for 30 seconds, or just until warm. Set aside. Preheat microwave browning dish at High as directed by manufacturer. Brush one side of swordfish steaks with oil mixture.

Place steaks, oiled-side-down, on preheated dish. Brush with remaining oil. Microwave at 70% (Medium High) for 3 minutes. Turn steaks over. Microwave at 70% (Medium High) for 4 to 5 minutes, or until fish flakes easily with fork, rotating dish once or twice.

Easy Crab & Mushroom Dinner

1 cup sliced fresh mushrooms
¼ cup chopped celery
2 tablespoons butter or margarine
2 tablespoons all-purpose flour
½ teaspoon salt
Dash cayenne

¾ cup milk
¼ cup sliced green onions
1 can (6 oz.) crab meat, rinsed, drained and cartilage removed
2 teaspoons sherry (optional)
Toasted French bread slices

4 to 6 servings

In 1-quart casserole, combine mushrooms, celery and butter. Cover. Microwave at High for 3½ to 5 minutes, or just until celery is tender-crisp, stirring once. Stir in flour, salt and cayenne. Blend in milk. Stir in onions. Microwave at High for 4 to 5½ minutes, or until mixture thickens and bubbles, stirring every 2 minutes.

Stir in crab meat and sherry. Microwave at High for 1 to 2 minutes, or until hot. Serve over French bread slices. Top with paprika or snipped fresh parsley, if desired.

Salmon-stuffed Green Pepper Rings

¼ cup chopped green pepper
¼ cup chopped onion
2 tablespoons butter or margarine
1 can (6¾ oz.) skinless, boneless salmon, drained
1 cup crushed herb-seasoned stuffing
1 egg, beaten
½ teaspoon Worcestershire sauce
4 green pepper rings (1 inch thick)
½ cup shredded Cheddar cheese
Dash cayenne

4 servings

In medium mixing bowl, combine chopped green pepper, onion and butter. Cover with plastic wrap. Microwave at High for 2 to 4 minutes, or until vegetables are tender, stirring once. Add salmon, stuffing, egg and Worcestershire sauce. Mix well.

Divide mixture into 4 equal portions. Press one-fourth of salmon mixture into the center of each pepper ring. Place rings in 9-inch square baking dish. Cover with plastic wrap. Microwave at 70% (Medium High) for 5 to 6 minutes, or until salmon mixture is firm and pepper rings are tender-crisp, rotating dish once or twice.

In small plastic food-storage bag, shake cheese and cayenne. Sprinkle one-fourth of cheese mixture over each pepper ring. Re-cover. Microwave at 70% (Medium High) for 1 to 2 minutes, or until cheese melts.

Tuna-stuffed Shells

⅓ cup chopped celery
⅓ cup shredded carrot
2 tablespoons butter or
   margarine
1 teaspoon instant chicken
   bouillon granules
⅛ teaspoon garlic powder
½ cup instant rice
½ cup hot water
1 can (6½ oz.) water-pack
   tuna, drained
1 can (10¾ oz.) condensed
   cream of mushroom soup
1 cup milk
8 uncooked jumbo pasta shells
1 hard-cooked egg, chopped
1 tablespoon snipped fresh
   parsley

4 servings

In 1-quart casserole, combine celery, carrot, butter, chicken bouillon granules and garlic powder. Cover. Microwave at High for 2 to 4 minutes, or until vegetables are tender, stirring once. Add rice and water. Re-cover. Microwave at High for 2 to 4 minutes, or until rice is tender and water is absorbed. Mix in tuna. Set aside.

In 9-inch round baking dish, combine soup and milk. Prepare pasta shells as directed on package. Rinse and drain. Stuff shells evenly with tuna mixture. Arrange stuffed shells in baking dish. Sprinkle with egg and parsley. Cover with plastic wrap. Microwave at 70% (Medium High) for 8 to 12 minutes, or until hot, rotating dish once or twice.

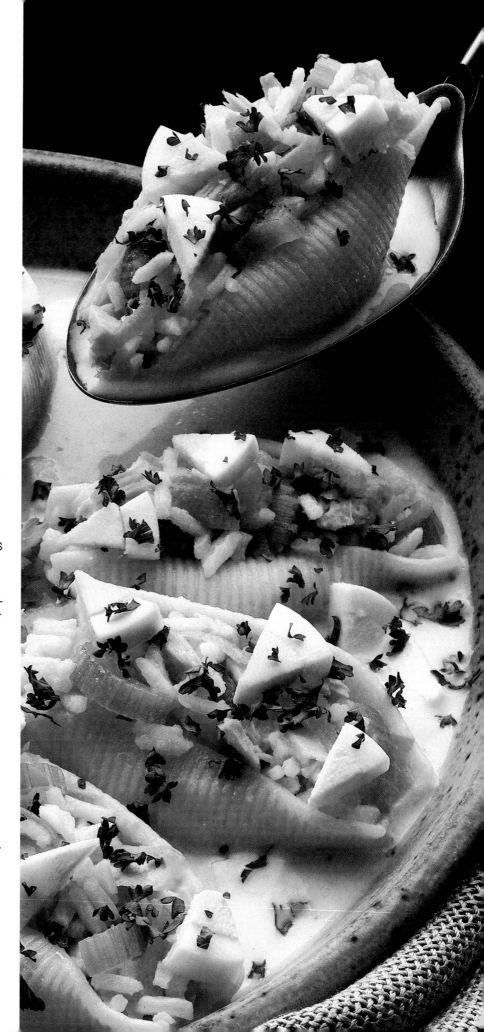

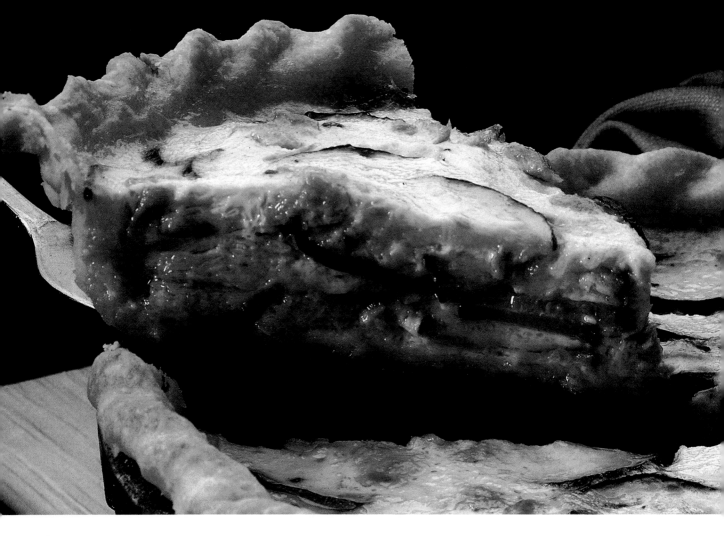

Salmon Brunch Pie

Crust:

- ¾ cup all-purpose flour
- 2 tablespoons grated Parmesan cheese
- ½ teaspoon salt
- ⅓ cup shortening
- 2 to 4 tablespoons cold water

Filling:

- 1½ cups thinly sliced zucchini
- 2 tablespoons butter or margarine
- ½ teaspoon garlic salt
- ¼ teaspoon dried oregano leaves
- ⅛ teaspoon pepper
- 2 tablespoons all-purpose flour
- ¾ cup milk
- 2 eggs, beaten
- 1 cup shredded Monterey Jack cheese
- 1 can (6¾ oz.) skinless, boneless salmon, drained

6 servings

How to Microwave Salmon Brunch Pie

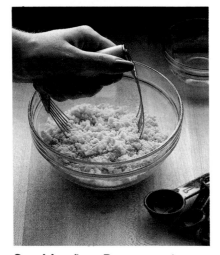

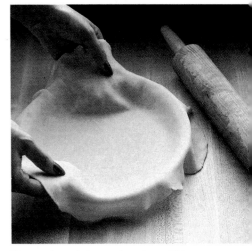

Combine flour, Parmesan cheese and salt in small mixing bowl. Cut in shortening to form coarse crumbs. Sprinkle with water, 1 tablespoon at a time, mixing with fork until particles are moistened and cling together. Form dough into ball. On lightly floured board, roll out dough at least 2 inches larger than inverted 9-inch pie plate.

Ease dough into pie plate. Trim and flute edges. Prick thoroughly. Microwave at High for 5 to 8 minutes, or until crust appears dry and opaque, rotating plate after every 2 minutes. Or preheat conventional oven to 400°F. Bake until light golden brown, 10 to 12 minutes. Set aside.

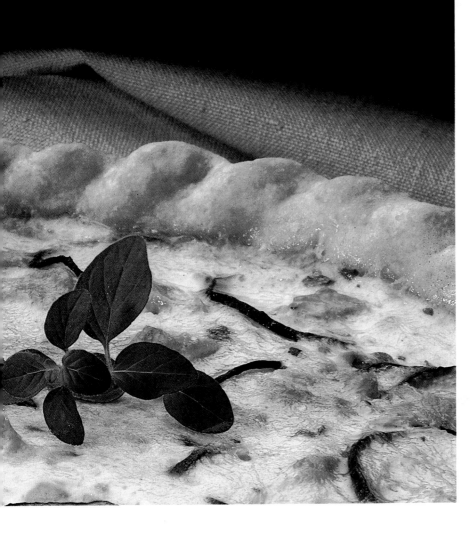

Seafood Platter with Lime Poppy Seed Dressing

½ lb. large shrimp, shelled and deveined
½ lb. sea scallops
½ lb. orange roughy fillet, about ½ to ¾ inch thick, cut into 1½-inch pieces
1 lime, cut in half
1 tablespoon butter or margarine
2 teaspoons all-purpose flour
1 teaspoon poppy seed
¾ teaspoon grated lime peel
¼ teaspoon salt
1 cup half-and-half
2 egg yolks, beaten
  Melon and apple wedges
  Seedless red and green grapes

4 to 6 servings

On 12-inch platter, arrange shrimp and scallops in single layer. Arrange fish on platter, with thinnest parts toward center of platter. Squeeze lime over shrimp, scallops and fish. Cover platter with plastic wrap. Microwave at 70% (Medium High) for 8 to 12 minutes, or until fish flakes easily with fork and shrimp and scallops are firm and opaque. Drain. Set aside, covered.

In 2-cup measure, microwave butter at High for 30 seconds to 1 minute, or until melted. Stir in flour, poppy seed, lime peel and salt. Blend in half-and-half. Microwave at High for 3 to 5 minutes, or until mixture thickens and bubbles, stirring every 2 minutes. Stir small amount of hot mixture gradually into egg yolks. Blend egg yolks back into hot mixture. Microwave at High for 30 seconds to 1½ minutes, or until mixture thickens slightly, stirring every 30 seconds. Do not overcook. Arrange fruit around seafood on platter. Serve with dressing.

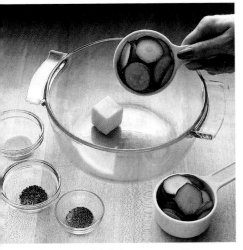

Combine zucchini, butter, garlic salt, oregano and pepper in 2-quart casserole. Cover. Microwave at High for 4 to 8 minutes, or until zucchini is tender, stirring once. Stir in flour. Blend in milk and eggs. Add remaining ingredients. Mix well.

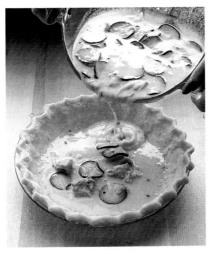

Pour mixture into prepared crust. Microwave at 50% (Medium) for 15 to 22 minutes, or until center of filling is set, rotating plate every 3 minutes. Let stand for 10 minutes.

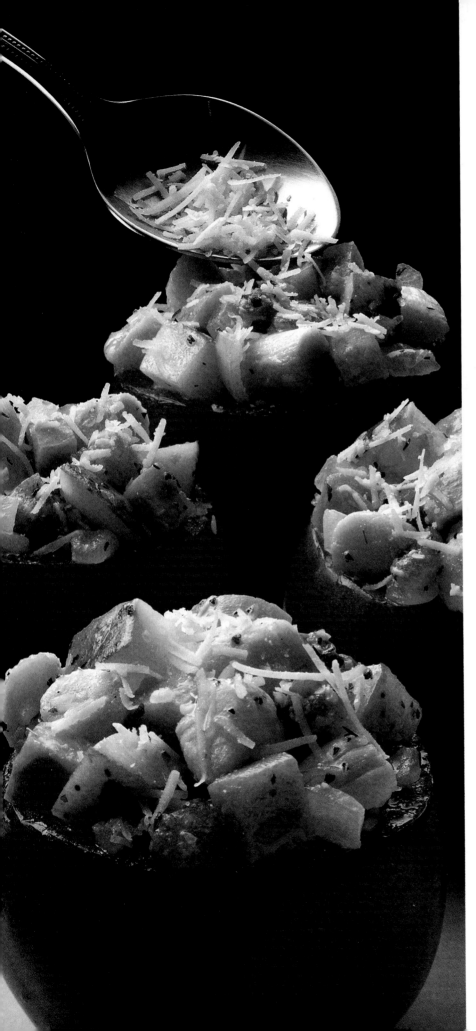

Garden Scallop Stuffed Tomatoes

 4 medium tomatoes
 ¾ cup cubed potato (½-inch cubes)
 ⅓ cup chopped carrot
 1 tablespoon butter or margarine
 ½ teaspoon dried bouquet garni seasoning
 ¾ lb. bay scallops
 ¼ cup chopped onion
 2 tablespoons grated Parmesan cheese
    Grated Parmesan cheese

4 servings

Remove and discard core from tomatoes. Cut thin slice from top of each tomato. Scoop out center pulp and seeds, discarding seeds. Chop pulp. Reserve ⅓ cup pulp. (Remainder may be reserved for use in other recipes.) Place tomato shells cut-side-down in colander to drain. Set aside.

In 1½-quart casserole, combine potato, carrot, butter and bouquet garni seasoning. Cover. Microwave at High for 2 to 4 minutes, or just until carrot and potato are tender-crisp, stirring once. Add scallops and onion. Mix well. Recover. Microwave at 70% (Medium High) for 4 to 8 minutes, or until scallops are firm and opaque, stirring once or twice. Drain.

Stir in 2 tablespoons Parmesan cheese and reserved ⅓ cup chopped tomato pulp. Spoon into tomato shells. Arrange stuffed tomatoes on platter. Sprinkle with additional Parmesan. Microwave at High for 3 to 7 minutes, or until tomatoes are warm, rotating platter once or twice.

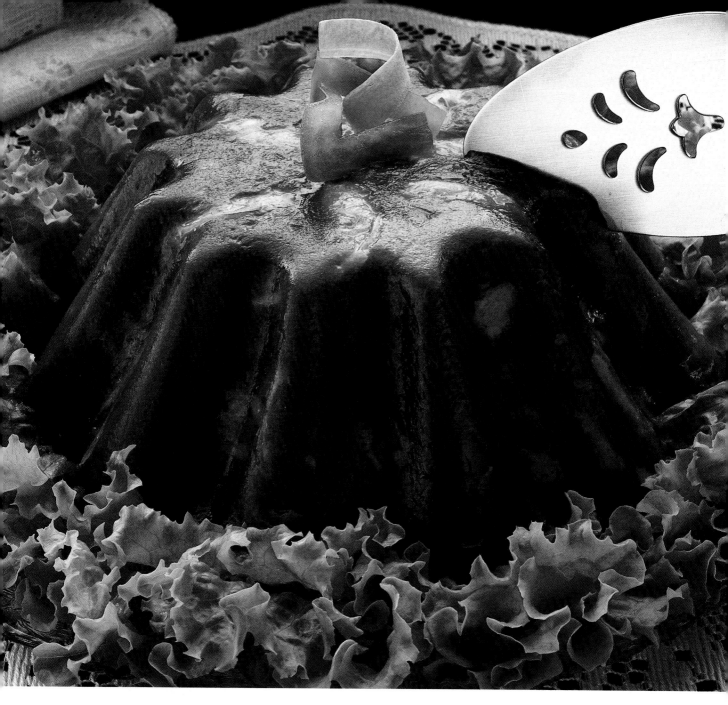

Shrimp & Fresh Vegetable Aspic

½ lb. large shrimp, shelled and deveined
1 envelope (.25 oz.) unflavored gelatin
1½ cups vegetable juice cocktail, divided
3 thin green pepper rings
3 thin yellow pepper rings
1 cup shredded carrots
1 cup thinly sliced celery
1 teaspoon Worcestershire sauce

4 servings

In 9-inch round baking dish, arrange shrimp in single layer. Cover with plastic wrap. Microwave at 70% (Medium High) for 5 to 8 minutes, or until shrimp are opaque, stirring once or twice. Drain. Let stand, covered, for 5 minutes. Rinse in cold water and drain.

In 2-cup measure, sprinkle gelatin over ½ cup vegetable juice cocktail. Let stand for 5 minutes. Lightly oil 1-quart mold. In prepared mold, layer shrimp, pepper rings, carrots and celery. Set aside. Microwave gelatin mixture at High for 1 to 2 minutes, or until gelatin dissolves.

Stir remaining 1 cup vegetable juice cocktail and the Worcestershire sauce into gelatin mixture. Pour evenly over layers in mold. Press top layer lightly, if necessary, to cover with gelatin mixture. Chill for 2 hours, or until set. Loosen edges. Invert mold onto serving platter. Garnish with leaf lettuce, if desired.

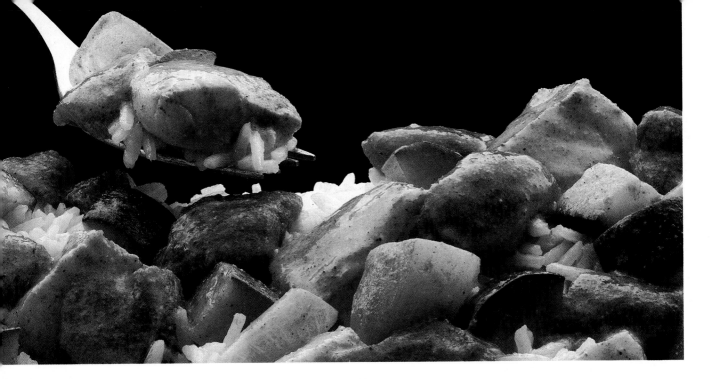

Curried Orange Roughy ▲ & Vegetables

1 small onion, cut into 1-inch pieces
1 tablespoon vegetable oil
1 tablespoon lemon juice
2 teaspoons curry powder
¼ teaspoon ground cinnamon
¼ teaspoon salt
⅛ teaspoon garlic powder
1 lb. orange roughy fillets, about ½ inch thick, cut into 1½-inch pieces
1 can (16 oz.) whole tomatoes, drained and cut up
1 small zucchini, cut into ½-inch cubes
Hot cooked rice

4 servings

In 2-quart casserole, place onion and vegetable oil. Cover. Microwave at High for 2 to 5 minutes, or until onion is tender. Add lemon juice, curry powder, cinnamon, salt and garlic powder. Mix well. Add fish pieces. Toss to coat.

Add tomatoes and zucchini. Re-cover. Microwave at 70% (Medium High) for 9 to 12 minutes, or until fish flakes easily with fork, stirring 2 or 3 times. Serve over hot cooked rice.

Linguine & Clam Bake

8 oz. uncooked linguine
2 tablespoons olive oil
⅓ cup snipped fresh parsley
2 cloves garlic, minced
1 teaspoon instant chicken bouillon granules
¼ teaspoon dried marjoram leaves
¼ teaspoon fresh ground pepper
2 tablespoons all-purpose flour
2 cans (6½ oz. each) minced clams, drained (reserve juice)
¼ cup milk
Grated Parmesan cheese

4 to 6 servings

Prepare linguine as directed on package. Rinse and drain. Set aside. In 2-quart casserole, combine olive oil, parsley, garlic, chicken bouillon granules, marjoram and pepper. Cover. Microwave at High for 3 to 4 minutes, or until garlic is tender. Stir in flour.

Blend in reserved clam juice and milk. Microwave at High for 3½ to 6 minutes, or until mixture thickens and bubbles, stirring 2 or 3 times. Stir in clams and cooked linguine. Cover. Microwave at High for 2 to 4 minutes, or until hot. Sprinkle with cheese before serving.

Saucy Creole Casserole

2 tablespoons olive oil
⅓ cup chopped green pepper
⅓ cup chopped celery
¼ cup chopped onion
1 can (16 oz.) whole tomatoes
1 can (15 oz.) tomato purée
1 pkg. (12 oz.) frozen uncooked large shrimp, shelled and deveined
1 cup instant rice
1 teaspoon chili powder
½ teaspoon sugar
¼ teaspoon dried oregano leaves
⅛ teaspoon garlic powder
⅛ teaspoon cayenne

4 to 6 servings

In 2-quart casserole, combine olive oil, green pepper, celery and onion. Cover. Microwave at High for 3 to 5 minutes, or until vegetables are tender, stirring once. Add whole tomatoes; stir to break apart.

Add remaining ingredients. Mix well. Re-cover. Microwave at 70% (Medium High) for 18 to 23 minutes, or until shrimp are opaque, stirring 2 or 3 times. Serve in bowls with French bread, if desired.

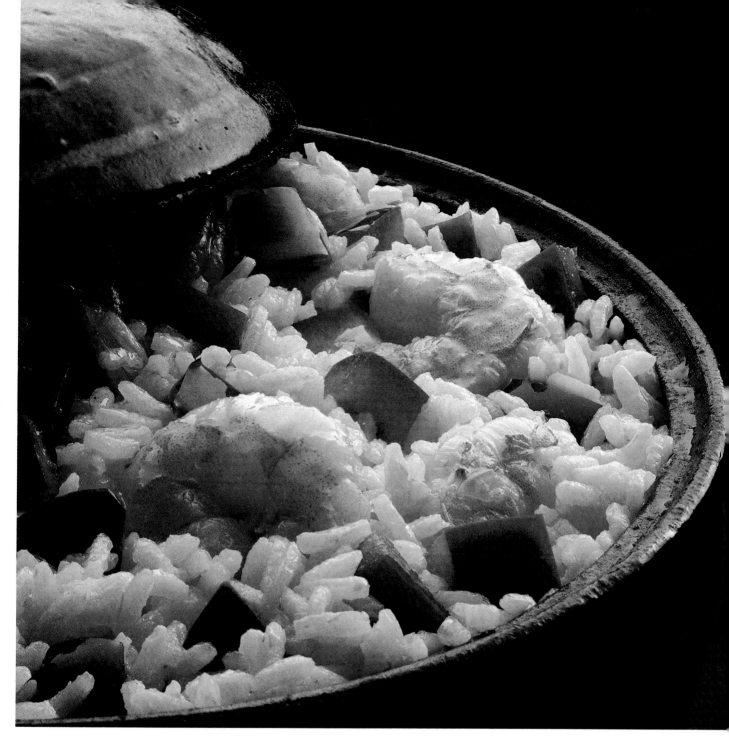

Saffron Shrimp & Tomatoes

1 cup uncooked long-grain white rice

1⅔ cups ready-to-serve chicken broth

⅓ cup milk

½ cup coarsely chopped green pepper

⅓ cup chopped onion

1 tablespoon olive oil (optional)

Dash ground saffron

½ lb. medium shrimp, shelled and deveined

1 medium tomato, seeded and coarsely chopped

4 to 6 servings

In 2-quart casserole, combine all ingredients, except shrimp and tomato. Mix well. Cover. Microwave at High for 8 minutes. Microwave at 50% (Medium) for 12 to 20 minutes longer, or until rice is tender and liquid is absorbed. Stir in shrimp. Re-cover. Microwave at High for 3 to 5 minutes, or until shrimp is opaque. Stir in tomato. Let stand, covered, for 2 minutes.

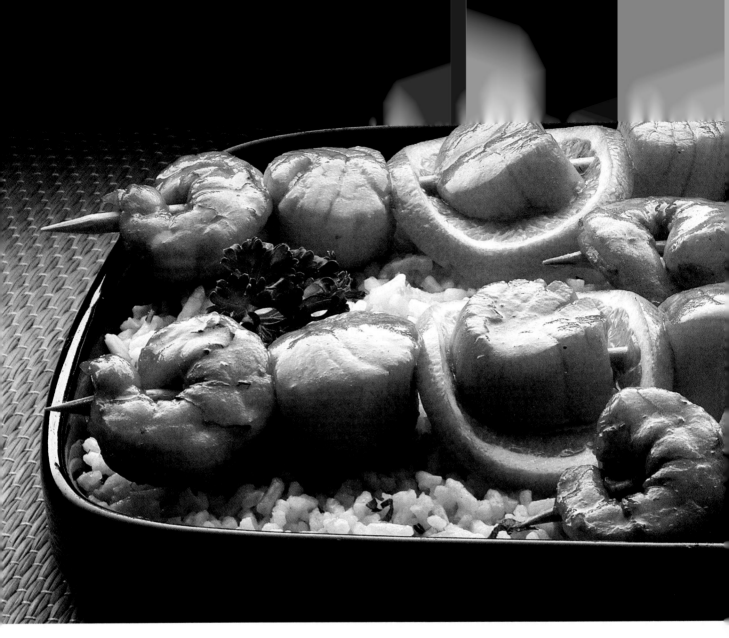

Oriental Orange Seafood Kabobs

- 3 tablespoons teriyaki sauce
- 1 tablespoon orange marmalade
- 12 sea scallops (about ½ lb.)
- 8 large shrimp (about ½ lb.), shelled and deveined
- 4 wooden skewers, 10-inch
- 4 thin orange slices
- 1 cup ready-to-serve chicken broth
- 1 tablespoon butter or margarine
- 1 teaspoon dried parsley flakes
- ¼ teaspoon grated orange peel
- 1 cup instant rice

4 servings

How to Microwave Oriental Orange Seafood Kabobs

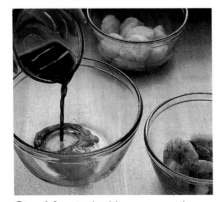

Combine teriyaki sauce and orange marmalade in medium mixing bowl. Microwave at High for 30 seconds to 1 minute, or until marmalade melts, stirring once. Add scallops and shrimp. Stir to coat. Let stand for 15 minutes.

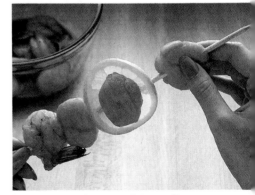

Place 1 shrimp and 1 scallop on skewer. Wrap 1 orange slice around 1 scallop and add to skewer. Add 1 more scallop and 1 more shrimp. Repeat sequence with remaining skewers.

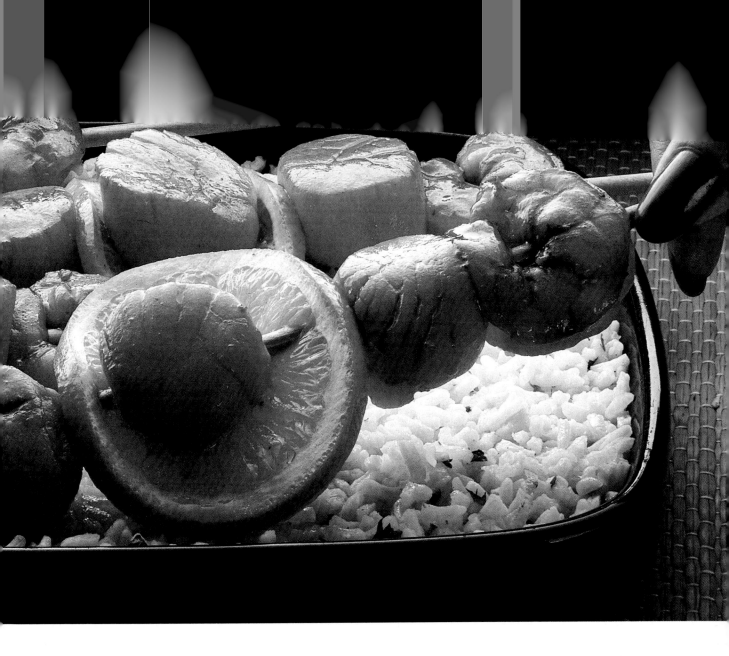

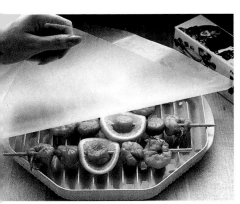

Arrange kabobs on roasting rack. Microwave at 70% (Medium High) for 9 to 11 minutes, or until shrimp and scallops are firm and opaque, rotating rack and rearranging kabobs twice. Cover with wax paper; let stand.

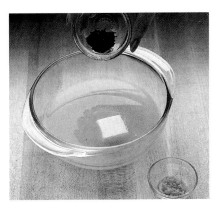

Combine broth, butter, parsley and orange peel in 1-quart casserole. Cover. Microwave at High for 4 to 5 minutes, or until broth boils.

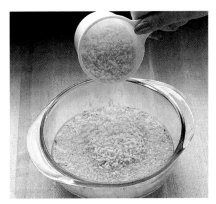

Stir in rice. Re-cover. Microwave at High for 1 minute. Let stand for 5 minutes, or until liquid is absorbed. Serve kabobs on rice.

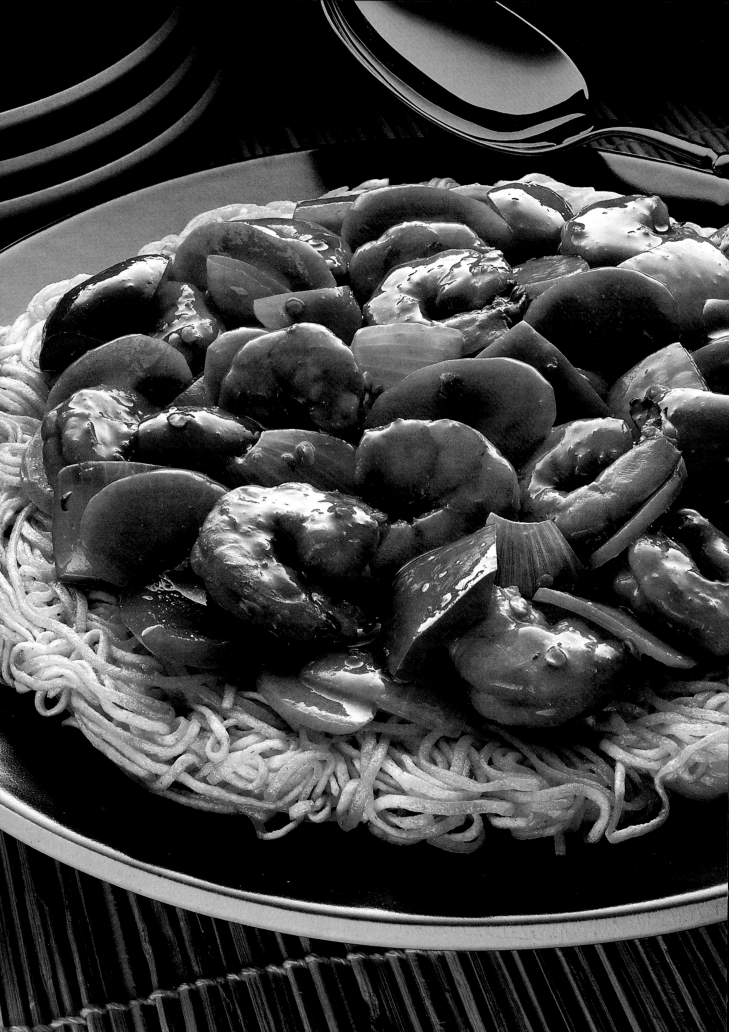

◀ Spicy Shrimp & Pan-fried Noodles

- 1 small onion, cut into 1-inch chunks
- ½ medium green pepper, cut into 1-inch chunks
- 1 medium carrot, thinly sliced
- 3 tablespoons vegetable oil, divided
- ¼ cup soy sauce
- ½ teaspoon sesame oil
- ¼ teaspoon crushed red pepper flakes
- ¾ teaspoon sugar
- 2 teaspoons cornstarch
- ¾ lb. large shrimp, shelled and deveined
- 8 oz. uncooked angel hair pasta

4 servings

In 2-quart casserole, combine onion, green pepper, carrot and 1 tablespoon vegetable oil. Cover. Microwave at High for 4 to 6 minutes, or until vegetables are tender-crisp, stirring once. Set aside.

In medium mixing bowl, combine soy sauce, sesame oil, red pepper flakes, sugar and cornstarch. Stir to dissolve cornstarch. Add shrimp. Toss to coat. Microwave at 70% (Medium High) for 7 to 10 minutes, or until shrimp are opaque and sauce is thickened and translucent, stirring once or twice. Add shrimp mixture to vegetable mixture. Cover to keep warm. Set aside.

Prepare pasta as directed on package. Rinse and drain. In 9-inch non-stick skillet, heat remaining 2 tablespoons vegetable oil conventionally over medium-high heat. Add pasta, pressing into an even layer. Cook for about 4 to 5 minutes, or until golden brown. Invert pasta onto serving plate, browned-side-up. If necessary, reheat shrimp mixture at 70% (Medium High) for 2 minutes. Top pasta with shrimp mixture.

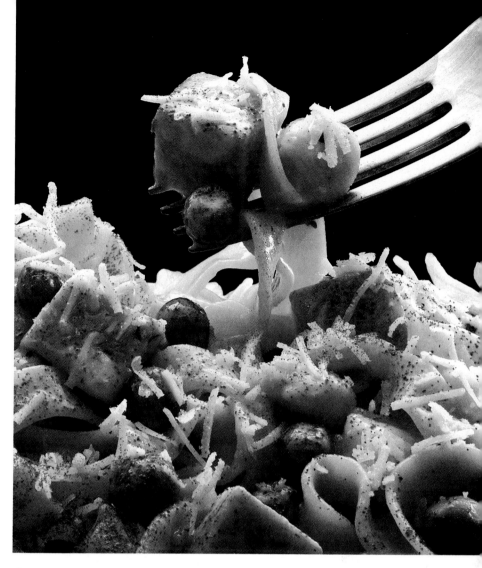

Scallop & Ham Bake ▲

- 1 cup ricotta or cottage cheese
- ⅓ cup milk
- 3 tablespoons grated Parmesan cheese
- ½ teaspoon dried marjoram leaves
- ¼ teaspoon salt
- 1 pkg.(10 oz.) frozen peas
- ½ lb. bay scallops
- 2 teaspoons lemon juice
- 1 teaspoon dried parsley flakes
- 3 cups uncooked egg noodles
- ½ cup cubed fully cooked ham (½-inch cubes)
- Grated Parmesan cheese
- Paprika

4 to 6 servings

In food processor or blender, combine ricotta cheese, milk, 3 tablespoons Parmesan cheese, the marjorarn and salt. Process until smooth. Set aside. Place peas in 1-quart casserole. Microwave at High for 4 to 5 minutes, or until defrosted. Drain. Set aside.

In 2-quart casserole, combine scallops, lemon juice and parsley. Cover. Microwave at 70% (Medium High) for 3½ to 6 minutes, or until scallops are firm and opaque. Drain. Set aside.

Prepare noodles as directed on package. Rinse and drain. Add noodles, peas and ham to scallops. Stir in ricotta mixture. Cover. Microwave at High for 4 minutes. Stir. Sprinkle with Parmesan cheese and paprika. Re-cover. Microwave at High for 2 to 6 minutes, or until hot.

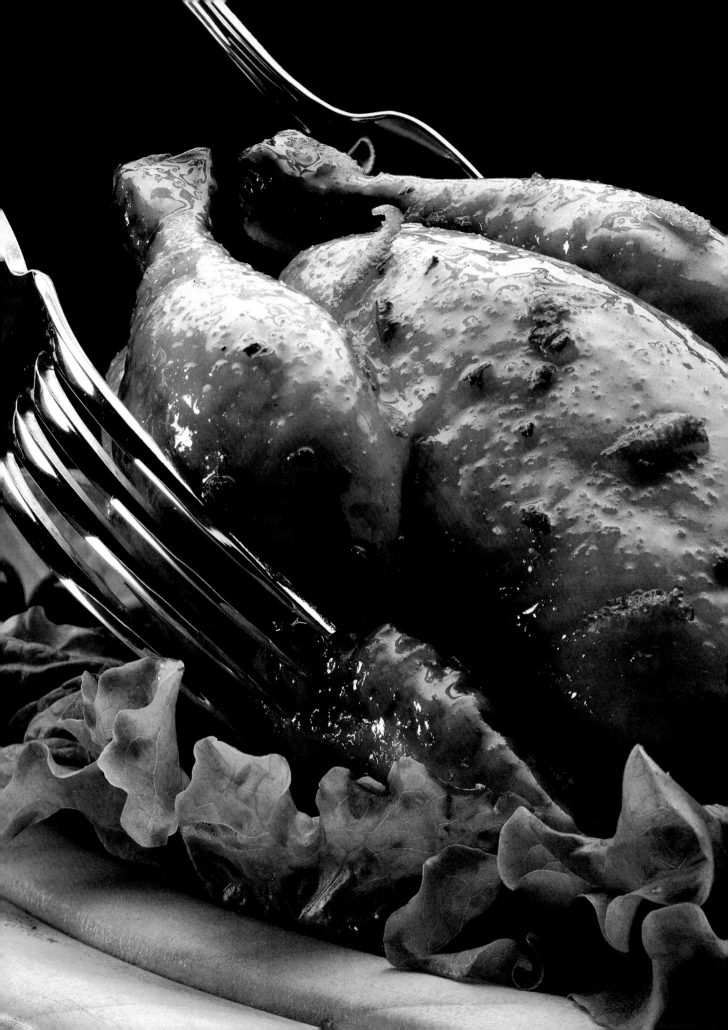

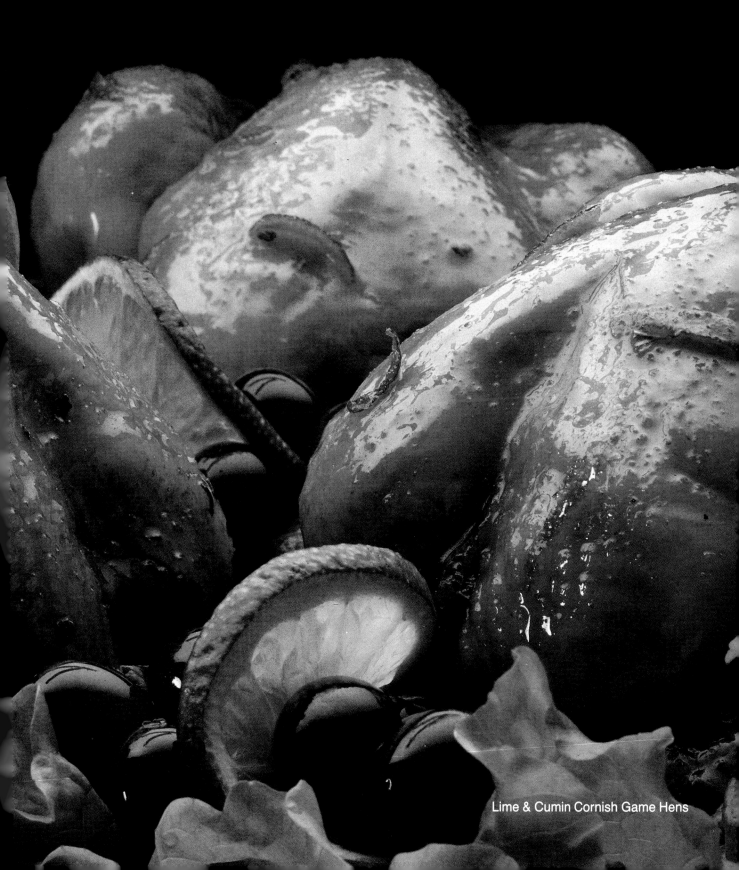

Lime & Cumin Cornish Game Hens

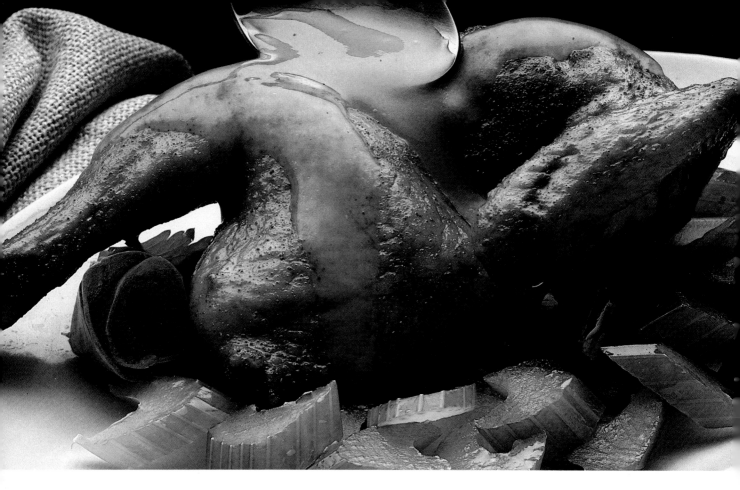

Savory Fruit-stuffed Cornish Game Hens

⅓ cup chopped celery
¼ cup pitted prunes, cut up
¼ cup dried apricots, cut up
2 tablespoons currants
2 tablespoons finely chopped onion
2 tablespoons butter or margarine
1 cup soft whole wheat bread crumbs
½ teaspoon poultry seasoning
¼ teaspoon salt
Dash pepper
2 Cornish game hens (24 oz. each)
Paprika

Sauce:
1 tablespoon cornstarch
¼ teaspoon salt
Dash pepper
¾ cup ready-to-serve chicken broth
¼ cup apricot nectar
¼ teaspoon bouquet sauce

4 servings

In 1-quart casserole, combine celery, prunes, apricots, currants, onion and butter. Cover. Microwave at High for 3 to 5 minutes, or until celery is tender-crisp, stirring once. Add bread crumbs, poultry seasoning, salt and pepper. Stir until moistened. Set aside.

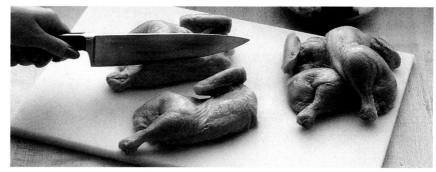

Split Cornish hens in half by cutting along breastbone and along each side of backbone. Discard backbone. Gently lift and loosen skin from breast area of each half. Place one-fourth of stuffing mixture under loosened skin. Secure with wooden picks.

Arrange breast-side-up in 10-inch square casserole. Sprinkle evenly with paprika. Cover with wax paper. Microwave at High for 16 to 20 minutes, or until legs move freely and juices run clear, rearranging once or twice. Set aside, covered.

In 2-cup measure, combine cornstarch, salt and pepper. Blend in broth, apricot nectar and bouquet sauce. Microwave at High for 4 to 5½ minutes, or until mixture is thickened and translucent, stirring 2 or 3 times. Serve sauce over Cornish hens.

Carrot-stuffed Chicken

Stuffing:

- ⅔ cup shredded carrot
- 1 tablespoon sliced green onion
- 2 teaspoons snipped fresh parsley
- 1 clove garlic, minced
- 2 tablespoons butter or margarine
- ⅓ cup seasoned dry bread crumbs
- ¼ teaspoon seasoned salt
- ¼ teaspoon dried marjoram leaves

2½ to 3-lb. whole broiler-fryer chicken

Butter Baste:

- 1 tablespoon butter or margarine
- ¼ teaspoon seasoned salt
- ¼ teaspoon paprika

4 servings

In 1-quart casserole, combine carrot, onion, parsley, garlic and 2 tablespoons butter. Cover. Microwave at High for 2 to 3 minutes, or until butter melts. Stir in remaining stuffing ingredients. Set aside.

Gently lift and loosen skin from breast area of chicken. Place stuffing mixture evenly under loosened skin. Secure with wooden picks. Secure legs together with string. Place breast-side-down on roasting rack. Set aside.

In small bowl, microwave butter at High for 45 seconds to 1 minute, or until melted. Stir in seasoned salt and the paprika. Brush half of butter mixture on chicken. Cover with wax paper. Microwave at High for 5 minutes. Turn chicken breast-side-up. Brush with remaining butter mixture. Re-cover. Microwave at High for 15 to 25 minutes, or until legs move freely and juices run clear, rotating rack twice. Let stand, covered, for 10 minutes before carving.

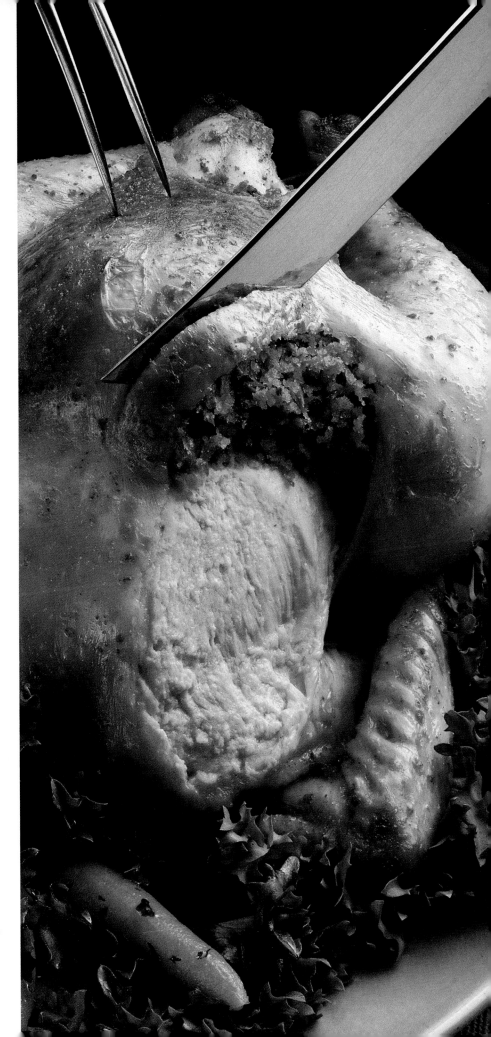

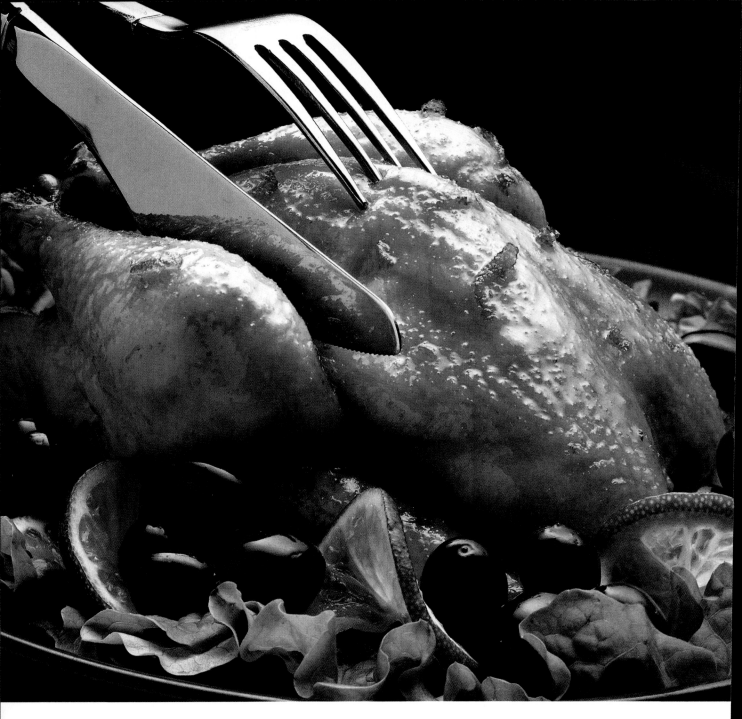

Lime & Cumin Cornish Game Hens

¼ cup dark corn syrup
2 tablespoons lime juice
½ to 1 teaspoon grated lime
   peel
1 teaspoon ground cumin,
   divided
½ teaspoon salt, divided
4 Cornish game hens
   (18 oz. each)
½ teaspoon dried oregano
   leaves
⅛ teaspoon pepper

In 1-cup measure, combine corn syrup, lime juice, lime peel, ½ teaspoon cumin and ¼ teaspoon salt. Microwave at High for 45 seconds to 1 minute, or until hot. Stir. Set aside. Secure hens' legs together with string. Place hens in large plastic food-storage bag. Pour corn syrup mixture over hens. Secure bag and place bag in dish. Refrigerate for at least 2 hours.

Remove hens from marinade and arrange breast-side-up on roasting rack. In small bowl, combine remaining ½ teaspoon cumin, ¼ teaspoon salt, the oregano and pepper. Rub mixture on hens. Microwave at High for 22 to 32 minutes, or until legs move freely and juices run clear, rotating rack twice. Let stand, covered, for 5 minutes.

4 servings

Raspberry Chicken

2 teaspoons cornstarch
¼ teaspoon onion salt
¼ teaspoon ground coriander, divided
 Dash ground allspice
1 tablespoon plus 1 teaspoon honey
2 teaspoons red wine vinegar
2 cups frozen unsweetened raspberries
2 bone-in whole chicken breasts (12 to 16 oz. each), split in half, skin removed
1 teaspoon dried parsley flakes
⅛ teaspoon pepper

4 servings

In 1-quart casserole, combine cornstarch, onion salt, ⅛ teaspoon coriander and the allspice. Blend in honey and vinegar. Mix well. Add raspberries. Cover. Microwave at High for 6 to 9 minutes, or until mixture is thickened and translucent, stirring 2 or 3 times. Set aside.

Arrange chicken breast halves on roasting rack, with meaty portions toward outside. In small bowl, combine remaining ⅛ teaspoon coriander, parsley and pepper. Mix well. Sprinkle evenly over chicken. Cover with wax paper. Microwave at High for 15 to 20 minutes, or until chicken near bone is no longer pink and juices run clear, rotating rack once or twice. Microwave raspberry sauce at High for 2 minutes, or until hot. Serve sauce over chicken.

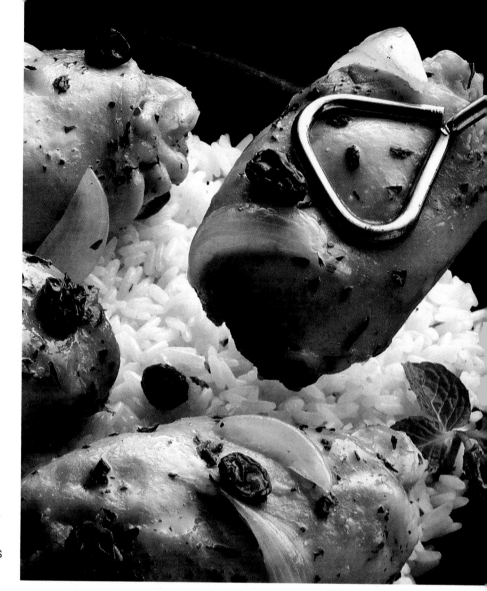

Orange-Mint Braised Chicken Thighs ▲

1 medium onion, cut into 8 wedges
2 tablespoons olive oil
2 teaspoons dried mint flakes
1 teaspoon grated orange peel
⅛ teaspoon cayenne
¼ cup ready-to-serve beef broth
¼ cup raisins
2 tablespoons white wine
½ teaspoon garlic salt
8 chicken thighs (about 3 lbs.), skin removed
 Hot cooked long-grain white or wild rice
 Orange slices (optional)

4 servings

In 1-quart casserole, combine onion, oil, mint, orange peel and cayenne. Cover. Microwave at High for 2 to 3 minutes, or until onion is tender-crisp, stirring once. Add broth, raisins, white wine and garlic salt. Mix well. Place chicken thighs in nylon cooking bag. Holding bag upright, add broth mixture. Shake bag gently to mix. Secure bag loosely with nylon tie or string. Refrigerate for at least 2 hours.

Place bag in 9-inch square baking dish. Microwave at High for 13 to 17 minutes, or until chicken near bone is no longer pink and juices run clear, carefully turning bag over twice. Let stand, closed, for 5 minutes. Serve chicken over rice. Garnish with orange slices.

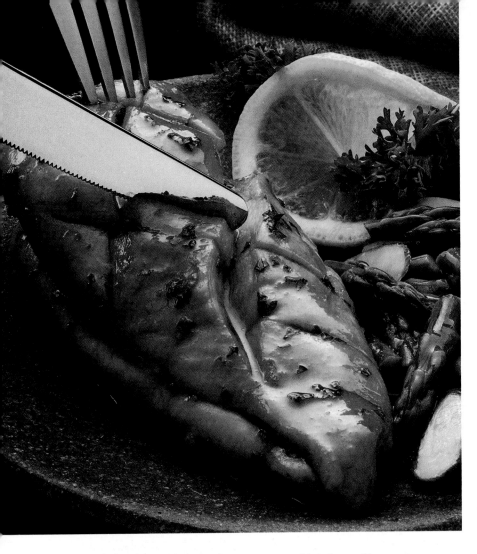

Honey Lemon Chicken Breasts

2 bone-in whole chicken breasts (12 to 16 oz. each), split in half, skin removed
2 tablespoons honey
1 tablespoon lemon juice
1 tablespoon packed brown sugar
1 tablespoon soy sauce
1 tablespoon snipped fresh parsley
¼ teaspoon bouquet sauce
¼ teaspoon grated lemon peel
4 thin lemon slices

4 servings

How to Microwave Honey Lemon Chicken Breasts

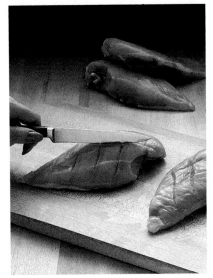

Score chicken breasts diagonally at 1-inch intervals, in diamond pattern, using a sharp knife. Set aside. In 9-inch square baking dish, combine remaining ingredients, except lemon slices. Stir to dissolve sugar.

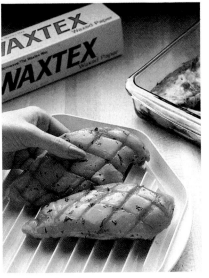

Add chicken breasts scored-side-down. Coat with honey mixture. Cover. Refrigerate for 30 minutes. Arrange breast halves scored-side-up on roasting rack, with meaty portions toward outside. Cover with wax paper.

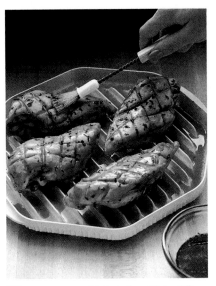

Microwave at High for 13 to 15 minutes, or until chicken near bone is no longer pink and juices run clear, rotating rack 2 or 3 times and basting with honey mixture once. Before serving, garnish with lemon slices.

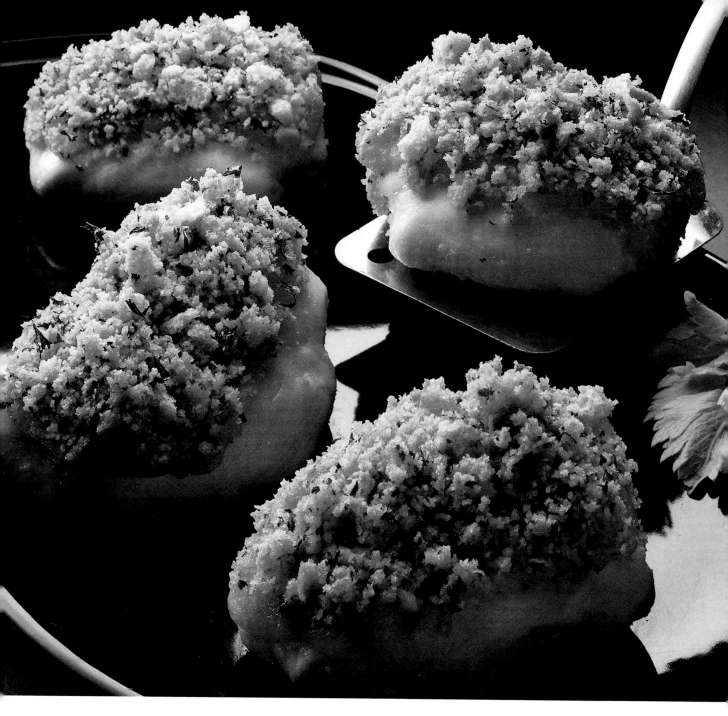

Golden Cheddary Chicken

2 boneless whole chicken breasts (12 to 16 oz. each), split in half, skin removed

4 slices Cheddar cheese (3 × 1 × ⅛-inch strips)

2 teaspoons butter or margarine

⅔ cup Cheddar cheese croutons, coarsely crushed

1½ teaspoons dried parsley flakes

⅛ teaspoon pepper

4 servings

Tuck thin ends under each chicken breast half to form a uniform shape. Arrange chicken in 9-inch square baking dish. Cover with wax paper. Microwave at High for 8 to 12 minutes, or until chicken is firm and no longer pink in center, rotating dish once. Place a strip of cheese over top of each chicken piece. Loosely cover with wax paper. Set aside.

In small mixing bowl, microwave butter at High for 30 seconds to 1 minute, or until melted. Stir in croutons, parsley and pepper. Sprinkle over cheese-topped chicken. Press lightly so crouton mixture adheres to cheese. Serve with long-grain white or wild rice, if desired.

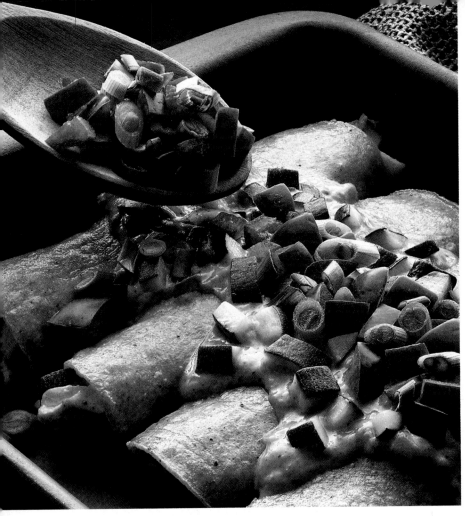

Chicken & Zucchini Enchiladas

¼ cup chopped onion
1 clove garlic, minced
1 tablespoon vegetable oil
1 tablespoon plus 2 teaspoons all-purpose flour
1 teaspoon chili powder
½ teaspoon ground cumin
½ teaspoon salt
1 cup milk
1½ cups cubed zucchini (¼-inch cubes), divided
1 cup cut-up cooked chicken
½ cup shredded Monterey Jack cheese
6 corn tortillas (6-inch)
Sliced green onion
Seeded chopped tomato

4 servings

In 2-quart casserole, combine chopped onion, garlic and oil. Cover. Microwave at High for 2 to 3 minutes, or until onion is tender. Stir in flour, chili powder, cumin and salt. Blend in milk. Microwave at High for 5 to 8 minutes, or until mixture thickens and bubbles, stirring every minute. Remove ½ cup sauce. Set aside. Add 1 cup cubed zucchini, the chicken and cheese to remaining sauce.

Soften tortillas as directed on package. Spoon ⅓ cup chicken mixture down center of each tortilla. Tightly roll up tortilla, enclosing filling. Arrange enchiladas seam-side-down in 9-inch square baking dish. Pour reserved sauce over top. Sprinkle with remaining ½ cup zucchini. Cover with plastic wrap. Microwave at 70% (Medium High) for 6 to 8 minutes, or until 140°F in center, rotating dish twice. Before serving, sprinkle with sliced green onion and chopped tomato.

Chili & Chicken Burritos

½ cup chopped onion
1 clove garlic, minced
1 lb. boneless whole chicken breast, skin removed, cut into 1-inch pieces
1 cup cooked white rice
1 cup seeded chopped tomato
1 can (4 oz.) chopped green chilies
1 cup shredded Cheddar cheese
¼ teaspoon dried oregano leaves
¼ teaspoon salt
4 flour tortillas (10-inch)
Shredded lettuce

Toppings:
Salsa or taco sauce
Guacamole
Green onions
Sour cream

4 servings

In 1-quart casserole, combine onion and garlic. Cover. Microwave at High for 2 to 3 minutes, or until onion is tender. Add chicken. Re-cover. Microwave at High for 4 to 6 minutes, or until chicken is no longer pink, stirring once. Mix in rice, tomato, chilies, cheese, oregano and salt. Set aside.

Place tortillas between 2 dampened paper towels. Microwave at High for 30 seconds to 1 minute, or just until tortillas feel warm. Spoon one-fourth of chicken mixture in center of each tortilla. Fold in one end of tortilla and then 2 sides. Roll to enclose filling. Place burritos seam-side-down in 9-inch square baking dish. Cover with dampened paper towel. Microwave at High for 6 to 7 minutes, or until burritos are hot, rotating dish once. Serve on shredded lettuce. Top as desired.

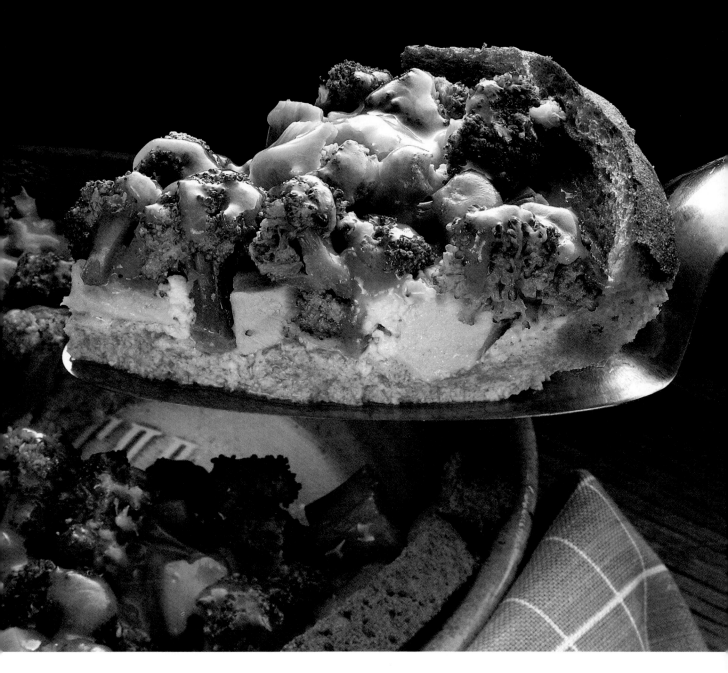

Whole Wheat Chicken & Broccoli Strata

1 pkg. (10 oz.) frozen
   chopped broccoli
4 to 5 slices whole wheat
   bread
1 cup cubed cooked chicken
   or turkey (½-inch cubes)
½ cup shredded Swiss cheese
1¼ cups milk
3 eggs, beaten
¾ teaspoon onion salt
½ teaspoon dry mustard
   Dash cayenne
½ cup shredded Cheddar
   cheese

6 servings

Unwrap broccoli and place on plate. Microwave at High for 4 to 6 minutes, or until defrosted. Drain. Set aside. Lightly grease a 10-inch pie plate. Cut each slice of bread in half diagonally. Fit bread halves around bottom and sides of pie plate, with crusts forming top edge. Top with chicken, Swiss cheese and broccoli. Set aside.

In 4-cup measure, blend milk, eggs, onion salt, mustard and cayenne. Pour evenly over broccoli mixture. Cover with plastic wrap. Refrigerate for at least 4 hours, or overnight.

Cover broccoli mixture with wax paper. Microwave at High for 5 minutes. Microwave at 70% (Medium High) for 15 to 28 minutes longer, or until knife inserted in center comes out clean, rotating pie plate twice. Sprinkle top with Cheddar cheese. Loosely cover with wax paper. Let stand for 5 minutes.

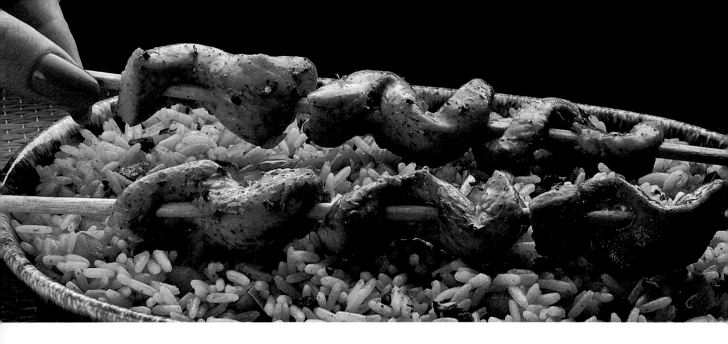

Spicy Rice & Skewered Chicken

1½ lbs. boneless whole chicken breasts, skin removed, cut into ½-inch strips
½ cup finely chopped onion, divided
1 tablespoon soy sauce
1 tablespoon packed brown sugar
1 tablespoon lemon juice

1 teaspoon chili powder, divided
⅓ cup chopped celery
¼ cup chopped green pepper
1 clove garlic, minced
1 tablespoon vegetable oil
2 tablespoons chopped pimiento

2 tablespoons snipped fresh parsley, divided
½ teaspoon salt
¼ teaspoon cayenne
1 cup uncooked long-grain white rice
2 cups hot water
6 wooden skewers, 10-inch

4 to 6 servings

How to Microwave Spicy Rice & Skewered Chicken

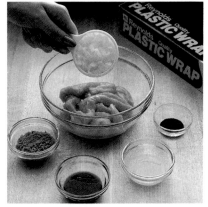

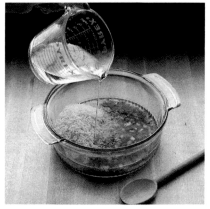

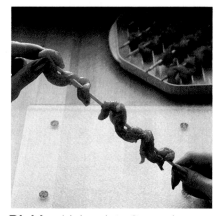

Combine chicken, ¼ cup onion, the soy sauce, brown sugar, lemon juice and ½ teaspoon chili powder in small mixing bowl. Mix well. Cover. Set aside. In 2-quart casserole, combine remaining ¼ cup onion, the celery, green pepper, garlic and oil. Cover. Microwave at High for 3 to 4 minutes, or until vegetables are tender, stirring twice.

Add remaining ½ teaspoon chili powder, the pimiento, 1 tablespoon parsley, the salt, cayenne, rice and water. Re-cover. Microwave at High for 5 minutes. Microwave at 50% (Medium) for 15 to 25 minutes longer, or until rice is tender and liquid is absorbed. Let stand, covered, for 5 minutes.

Divide chicken into 6 equal portions. Thread 1 portion loosely onto each skewer. Arrange skewers on roasting rack. Cover with wax paper. Microwave at High for 5 to 7 minutes, or until chicken is no longer pink, turning over and rearranging skewers twice. Serve skewered chicken on rice. Before serving, sprinkle with remaining parsley.

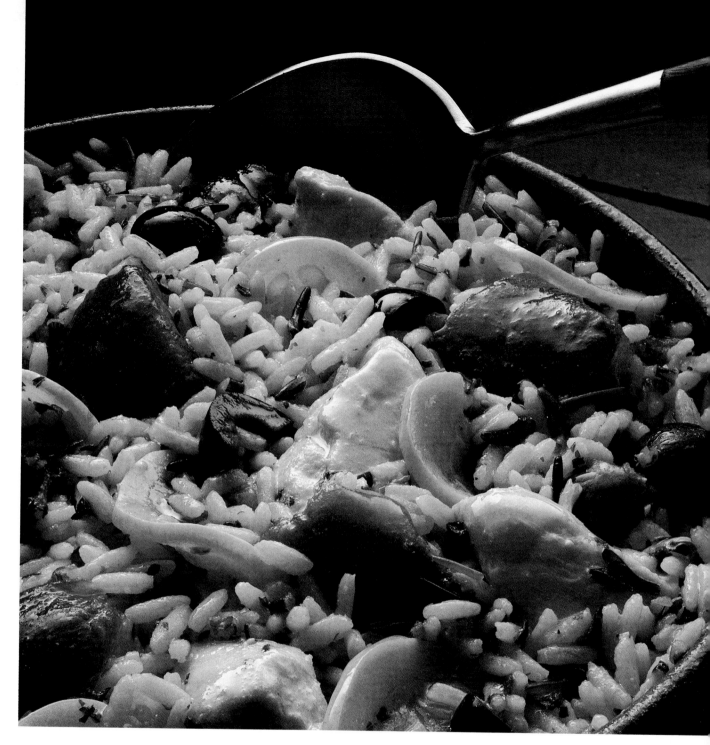

Warm Spanish Chicken Salad

1 lb. boneless whole chicken breast, skin removed, cut into ¾-inch cubes

1 pkg. (6 oz.) seasoned long-grain white and wild rice mix

2 cups water

1 small summer squash, cut in half lengthwise and thinly sliced

1 medium tomato, peeled, seeded and cut into chunks

⅓ cup quartered pitted black olives

3 tablespoons olive oil

1 tablespoon lemon juice

1 tablespoon red wine vinegar

6 servings

In 2-quart casserole, combine chicken, rice and seasoning packet, and water. Stir. Cover. Microwave at High for 5 minutes. Microwave at 50% (Medium) for 30 to 35 minutes longer, or until rice is tender and liquid is absorbed. Stir in squash. Re-cover. Let stand for 5 minutes. Add remaining ingredients. Mix well. Serve with a slotted spoon.

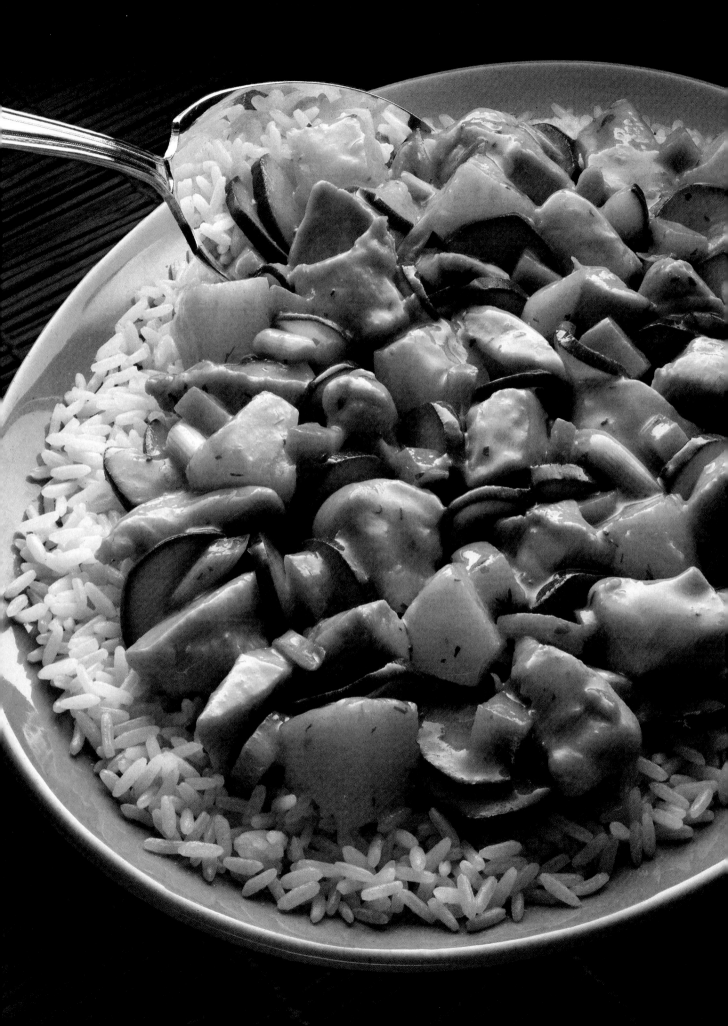

◄ Caribbean Chicken Medley

1 tablespoon cornstarch
½ teaspoon dry mustard
½ teaspoon ground ginger
½ teaspoon dried cilantro leaves
1 can (8 oz.) pineapple chunks
   in juice, drained (reserve
   ¼ cup juice)
2 tablespoons soy sauce
2 tablespoons Russian
   dressing or catsup

1½ lbs. boneless whole chicken
   breasts, skin removed, cut
   into 1-inch pieces
1 small zucchini, cut in half
   lengthwise and thinly sliced
¼ cup chopped carrot
6 green onions, sliced
   diagonally (½-inch slices)

6 servings

In 2-quart casserole, combine cornstarch, mustard, ginger and cilantro. Blend in ¼ cup pineapple juice, the soy sauce and dressing. Add chicken, zucchini and carrot. Cover. Microwave at High for 10 to 14 minutes, or until sauce is thickened and translucent, stirring 3 times. Stir in onions and pineapple chunks. Re-cover. Microwave at High for 2 minutes, or until hot. Serve over hot cooked rice, if desired.

Chicken Almond Ding

1 lb. boneless whole chicken
   breast, skin removed, cut
   into ½-inch cubes
2 teaspoons soy sauce
2 teaspoons cornstarch
2 teaspoons vegetable oil,
   divided
¼ teaspoon sesame oil
¼ teaspoon salt
⅛ teaspoon garlic powder

½ cup whole blanched
   almonds
½ cup ready-to-serve chicken
   broth
1½ cups thinly sliced celery
2 tablespoons sliced green
   onion
2 oz. fresh pea pods, cut into
   ½-inch lengths
   Hot cooked rice

4 servings

In 2-quart casserole, combine chicken, soy sauce, cornstarch, 1 teaspoon vegetable oil, the sesame oil, salt and garlic powder. Mix well. Let stand at room temperature for 15 minutes. In 9-inch pie plate, place remaining 1 teaspoon vegetable oil and the almonds. Toss to coat. Microwave at High for 5 to 10 minutes, or until almonds are golden brown, stirring after every 2 minutes. Set aside.

Microwave chicken mixture at High for 3 to 4 minutes, or just until chicken is no longer pink, stirring once. Add broth. Mix well. Add celery and onion. Cover. Microwave at High for 6 to 9 minutes, or until sauce is thickened and translucent and celery is tender. Add almonds and pea pods. Microwave at High for 1 minute. Let stand, covered, for 5 minutes. Serve with rice.

Lemon Chicken & Broccoli with Poppy Seed Noodles

1 lb. boneless whole chicken
   breast, skin removed, cut
   into ½-inch strips
1 tablespoon plus 2 teaspoons
   vegetable oil, divided
1 tablespoon sliced green
   onion
1½ teaspoons grated lemon
   peel, divided
1 teaspoon vinegar
¼ teaspoon sugar
1 pkg. (10 oz.) frozen chopped
   broccoli or 2 cups fresh
   broccoli flowerets
2 tablespoons water
2 tablespoons butter or
   margarine
1 teaspoon poppy seed
¼ teaspoon salt
8 oz. uncooked wide egg
   noodles

4 servings

In 2-quart casserole, combine chicken strips, 2 teaspoons oil, the onion, ½ teaspoon lemon peel, the vinegar and sugar. Mix well. Set aside. In 1½-quart casserole, combine broccoli and water. Cover. Microwave at High for 4 to 6 minutes, or until broccoli is hot, stirring once to break apart. Drain. Set aside.

In 1-cup measure, microwave butter at High for 45 seconds to 1 minute, or until melted. Add remaining 1 tablespoon oil and 1 teaspoon lemon peel, the poppy seed and salt. Prepare egg noodles as directed on package. Rinse and drain. Toss cooked noodles with butter mixture. Cover to keep warm. Set aside.

Microwave chicken mixture at High for 4 to 5½ minutes, or until chicken is no longer pink, stirring once or twice. Add broccoli to chicken mixture. Arrange noodles on serving platter. Top with chicken and broccoli mixture. Garnish with lemon slices, if desired.

Roast Turkey with Garden Squash Stuffing

1 small onion, sliced
1 clove garlic, minced
1 teaspoon dried basil leaves
½ teaspoon dried thyme
   leaves
¼ teaspoon paprika
¼ teaspoon pepper
7½ to 8½-lb. bone-in turkey
   breast

Stuffing:

1 cup cubed zucchini
   (½-inch cubes)
1 cup cubed summer squash
   (½-inch cubes)
½ cup chopped onion
3 tablespoons butter or
   margarine
¼ teaspoon dried basil leaves
⅛ teaspoon dried thyme
   leaves
2 cups herb-seasoned
   stuffing mix
¼ to ⅓ cup ready-to-serve
   chicken broth
¼ teaspoon salt
   Dash pepper

10 to 12 servings

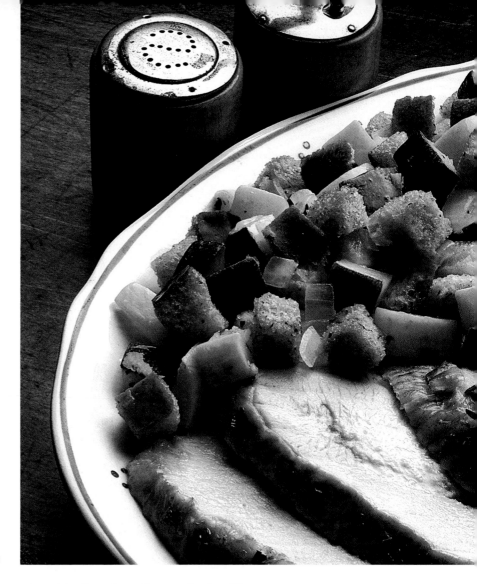

How to Microwave Roast Turkey with Garden Squash Stuffing

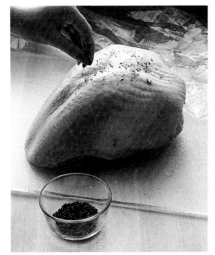

Place onion and garlic in nylon cooking bag. Set aside. In small dish, combine 1 teaspoon basil, ½ teaspoon thyme, the paprika and ¼ teaspoon pepper. Sprinkle evenly over turkey breast.

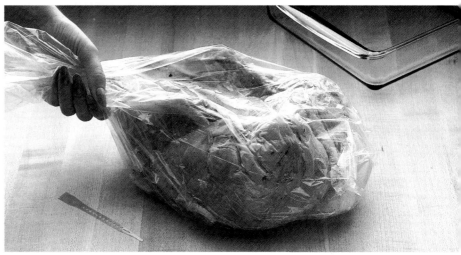

Place turkey skin-side-down in bag. Secure bag loosely with nylon tie or string. Place bag in 9-inch square baking dish. Estimate total cooking time at 12½ to 16½ minutes per pound, and divide total cooking time into 2 parts. Microwave at High for first 5 minutes. Microwave at 50% (Medium) for remainder of first half of time, rotating dish once.

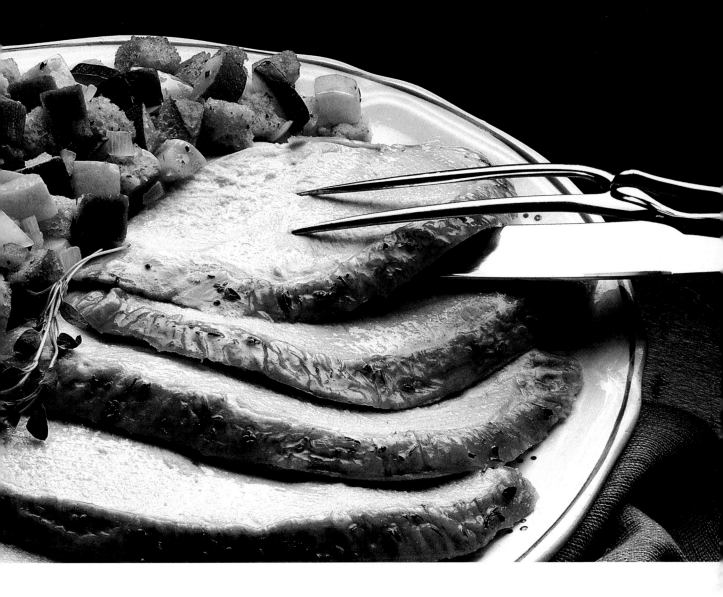

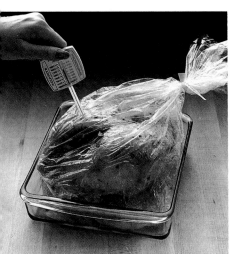

Turn turkey skin-side-up. Microwave at 50% (Medium) for second half of time, or until internal temperature registers 170°F in several places, rotating dish once. Let bag stand, closed, for 10 to 20 minutes before carving turkey.

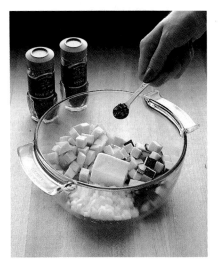

Combine zucchini, summer squash, onion, butter, basil and thyme leaves in 1½-quart casserole. Cover. Microwave at High for 5 to 7 minutes, or until vegetables are tender-crisp, stirring once.

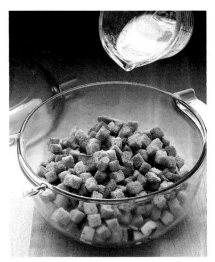

Add stuffing mix. Add enough broth to moisten. Stir in salt and pepper. Re-cover. Microwave at High for 3 minutes, or until hot. Serve with turkey.

Cranberry-stuffed Turkey Tenderloins

¾ cup frozen chopped
    cranberries, divided
½ cup sliced fresh mushrooms
¼ cup finely chopped onion
2 tablespoons plus 1 teaspoon
    packed brown sugar, divided
1 tablespoon dried parsley
    flakes, divided
½ teaspoon grated orange peel,
    divided
¼ teaspoon salt, divided
1 tablespoon butter or
    margarine
2 turkey tenderloins, (about
    ¾ lb. each)
⅓ cup orange juice
2 teaspoons cornstarch

4 to 6 servings

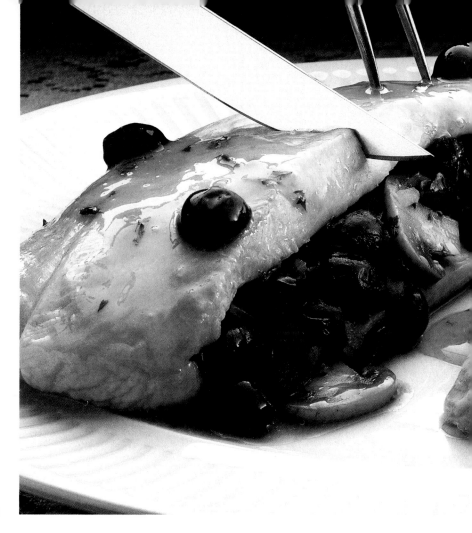

How to Microwave Cranberry-stuffed Turkey Tenderloins

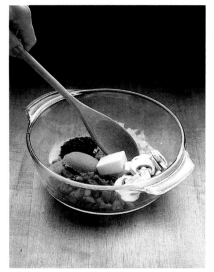

Combine ½ cup cranberries, the mushrooms, onion, 2 tablespoons brown sugar, 2 teaspoons parsley, ¼ teaspoon orange peel, ⅛ teaspoon salt and the butter in 1-quart casserole. Cover. Microwave at High for 2 to 3 minutes, or until mushrooms are tender, stirring once. Set aside.

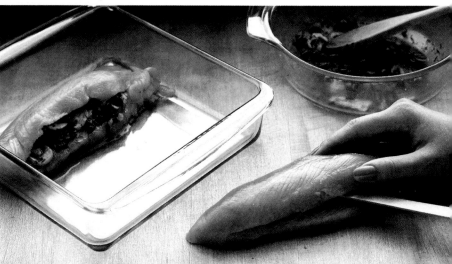

Slit each tenderloin lengthwise to within ½ inch of edge to form pocket. Fill each tenderloin with half of cranberry mixture. Arrange in 9-inch square baking dish, with opening toward center. Cover with wax paper. Microwave at 70% (Medium High) for 15 to 21 minutes, or until turkey is firm and no longer pink, rotating dish twice. Remove tenderloins to platter. Cover with foil to keep warm. Reserve cooking liquid.

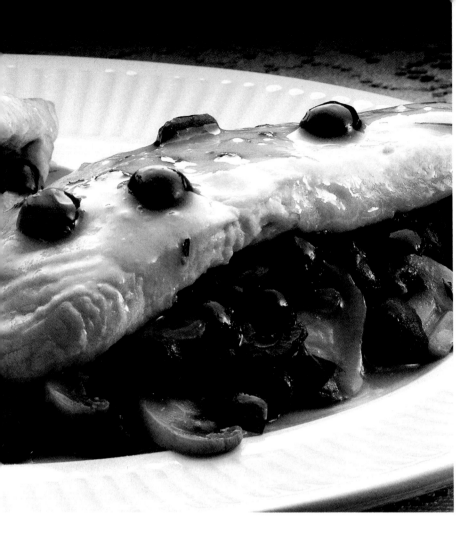

Fresh Fruit-stuffed Turkey

3- lb. boneless turkey breast

Stuffing:
½ cup chopped apple
½ cup chopped pear
½ small orange, peeled and
    chopped
¼ cup raisins
½ teaspoon ground cinnamon
⅛ teaspoon ground allspice
⅓ cup corn bread stuffing mix

2 teaspoons packed brown
    sugar
¼ teaspoon ground cinnamon

6 to 8 servings

Remove netting from turkey. Open turkey breast, separating breast halves. Place turkey skin-side-down. If necessary, cut slightly so breast lies flat, being careful not to cut all the way through. Set aside.

Combine all stuffing ingredients in medium mixing bowl. Mix well. Pack stuffing mixture down center of turkey breast. Reassemble breast, enclosing stuffing. Tie securely with string. In small bowl, combine brown sugar and cinnamon. Rub breast with brown sugar mixture.

Place breast skin-side-up in nylon cooking bag. Secure bag loosely with nylon tie or string. Place bag in 9-inch square baking dish. Microwave at 70% (Medium High) for 30 to 40 minutes, or until temperature registers 175°F in several places, rotating dish 2 or 3 times. Let stand, closed, for 10 minutes before slicing.

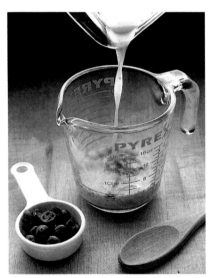

Place orange juice in 2-cup measure. Stir in cornstarch, remaining 1 teaspoon brown sugar, 1 teaspoon parsley, ¼ teaspoon orange peel and ⅛ teaspoon salt. Mix well.

Blend in reserved cooking liquid. Stir in remaining ¼ cup cranberries. Microwave at High for 3 to 4½ minutes, or until sauce is thickened and translucent, stirring twice. Serve sauce over turkey.

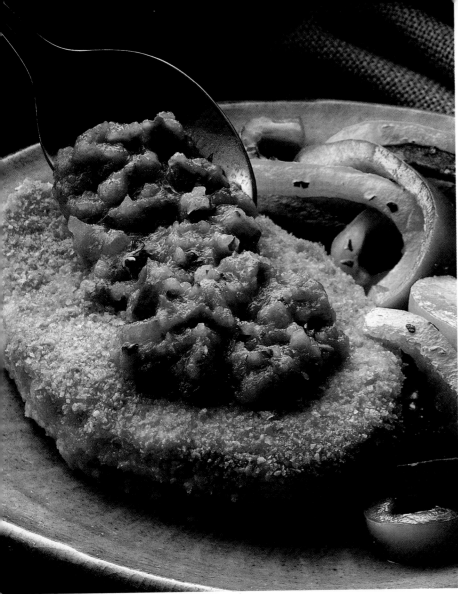

Turkey Cutlets with Green Chili Sauce

½ cup shredded Monterey Jack cheese

½ teaspoon ground cumin, divided

½ cup cornflake crumbs

⅛ teaspoon garlic powder

8 turkey cutlets (2 oz. each), about ¼ inch thick

Sauce:

1 can (4 oz.) chopped green chilies

¼ cup seeded chopped tomato

1 tablespoon snipped fresh parsley

½ teaspoon olive oil

¼ teaspoon salt

4 servings

In small bowl, combine cheese and ¼ teaspoon cumin. Set aside. In shallow dish, combine cornflake crumbs, garlic powder and remaining ¼ teaspoon cumin. Set aside.

Top each of 4 cutlets with one-fourth of cheese mixture, spreading to within ¼ inch of edge. Top with remaining cutlets, pressing edges gently together to seal. Dip stuffed cutlets in cornflake crumb mixture, pressing lightly to coat both sides.

Arrange cutlets on roasting rack. Microwave at 70% (Medium High) for 10 to 14 minutes, or until turkey is firm and no longer pink, rotating rack once or twice. Cover with wax paper to keep warm.

Place chopped green chilies in food processor or blender. Process until smooth. Add remaining sauce ingredients. Stir to combine. Serve cutlets topped with sauce.

Olive-topped Turkey Cutlets

1 lb. turkey cutlets, about ¼ inch thick

½ cup diagonally sliced celery (½-inch slices)

8 small pimiento-stuffed green olives, cut in half

8 medium pitted black olives, cut in half

1 clove garlic, minced

¼ cup white wine

1 tablespoon olive oil

1 tablespoon snipped fresh parsley

1 teaspoon instant chicken bouillon granules

1 teaspoon lemon juice

¼ teaspoon dried rubbed sage leaves

⅛ teaspoon pepper

4 to 6 servings

Arrange cutlets in 9-inch square baking dish. Top with celery, green and black olives and garlic. Set aside. In 1-cup measure, combine remaining ingredients. Mix well. Pour over cutlets. Cover with wax paper. Marinate at room temperature for 15 minutes. Cover. Microwave at 70% (Medium High) for 9 to 15 minutes, or until turkey is firm and no longer pink, rearranging once or twice.

Turkey Fajitas

Marinade:

- 1 tablespoon lemon juice
- 1 tablespoon white wine
- 1 tablespoon vegetable oil
- 1 tablespoon sliced green onion
- 1 teaspoon soy sauce
- 1 teaspoon packed brown sugar
- 1 clove garlic, minced
- ¼ teaspoon crushed red pepper flakes
- 2 drops liquid smoke flavoring

- ¾ lb. turkey tenderloin, cut into thin strips
- ½ medium green pepper, cut into thin strips
- ½ medium onion, thinly sliced
- 4 flour tortillas (8-inch)

Toppings:

- Salsa sauce
- Guacamole
- Seeded chopped tomato

4 servings

In 1½-quart casserole, combine all marinade ingredients. Add turkey strips. Stir to coat. Cover. Refrigerate for 30 minutes. Add green pepper and onion to marinated turkey. Re-cover. Microwave at 70% (Medium High) for 6 to 11 minutes, or until turkey is firm and no longer pink, stirring 3 times.

Place tortillas between 2 dampened paper towels. Microwave at High for 30 seconds to 1 minute, or just until tortillas feel warm. Spoon one-fourth of turkey, onion and green pepper mixture down the center of each tortilla. Top as desired. Roll up tortillas to enclose filling.

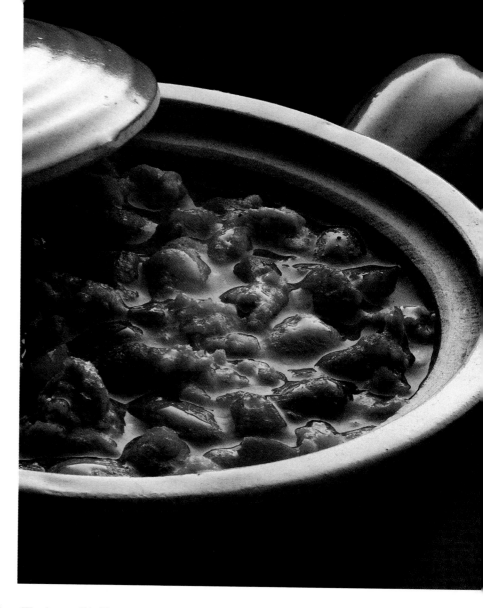

Turkey Chili ▲

- 1 cup chopped green pepper
- ½ cup chopped onion
- 1 clove garlic, minced
- 1 lb. ground turkey
- 1 can (28 oz.) whole tomatoes, cut up
- 1 can (16 oz.) pinto beans, drained
- 1 can (15 oz.) kidney beans, drained
- 1 can (10¾ oz.) condensed tomato soup
- ½ cup water
- 1 tablespoon plus 1 teaspoon chili powder
- ¾ teaspoon celery salt
- ¼ teaspoon cayenne
- ¼ teaspoon pepper

6 to 8 servings

In 3-quart casserole, combine green pepper, onion and garlic. Cover. Microwave at High for 2 minutes. Crumble ground turkey over vegetables. Re-cover. Microwave at High for 4 to 7 minutes, or until turkey is firm, stirring twice to break apart.

Add remaining ingredients. Mix well. Cover with wax paper. Microwave at High for 20 to 30 minutes, or until flavors blend, stirring 2 or 3 times. Let stand, covered, for 10 minutes. Top each serving with shredded Cheddar cheese, if desired.

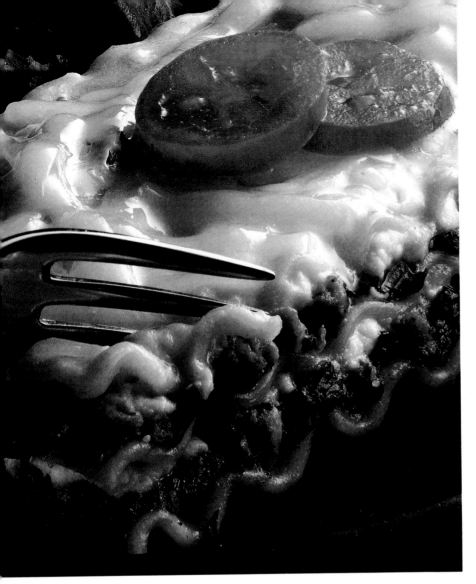

Mediterranean Lasagna

- 9 uncooked lasagna noodles
- 1 pkg. (10 oz.) frozen chopped spinach
- ½ lb. ground turkey
- 2 teaspoons instant minced onion
- 2 teaspoons snipped fresh parsley
- ½ teaspoon dried oregano leaves
- ½ teaspoon lemon pepper seasoning
- ¼ teaspoon ground cinnamon
- ½ teaspoon salt

Sauce:

- 2 tablespoons butter or margarine
- 2 tablespoons all-purpose flour
- 2 teaspoons snipped fresh parsley
- ¼ teaspoon salt
  Dash pepper
- 1¼ cups milk

- 1 cup ricotta cheese
- 1 cup shredded Monterey Jack cheese, divided
- 1 egg, beaten

6 servings

How to Microwave Mediterranean Lasagna

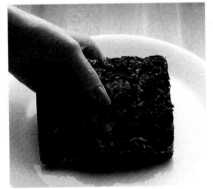

Prepare lasagna noodles according to package directions. Rinse and drain. Place noodles flat on plastic wrap. Set aside. Unwrap spinach and place on plate. Microwave at High for 4 to 6 minutes, or until defrosted. Drain, pressing to remove excess moisture. Set aside.

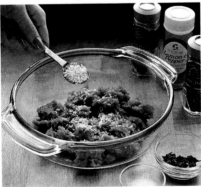

Crumble ground turkey into 1½-quart casserole. Add onion, 2 teaspoons parsley, the oregano, lemon pepper, cinnamon and ½ teaspoon salt. Cover. Microwave at High for 2 to 4 minutes, or until turkey is firm, stirring once to break apart. Mix in spinach. Set aside.

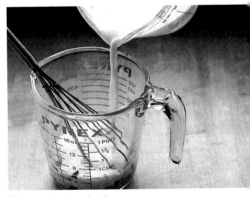

Place butter in 2-cup measure. Microwave at High for 45 seconds to 1 minute, or until melted. Stir in flour, parsley, salt and pepper. Blend in milk. Microwave at High for 3½ to 5 minutes, or until mixture thickens and bubbles, stirring 2 or 3 times. Stir ¾ cup sauce into meat mixture. Reserve remaining sauce.

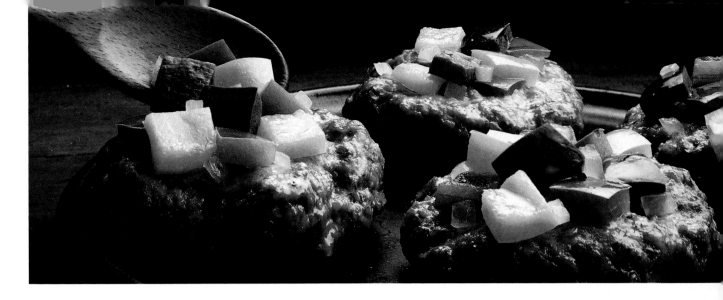

Italian Turkey Patties

1 cup green, red or yellow pepper chunks (¾-inch chunks)
¼ cup chopped onion
2 tablespoons Italian dressing
1 lb. ground turkey
1 egg, beaten
2 tablespoons seasoned dry bread crumbs
2 teaspoons snipped fresh parsley
¼ teaspoon Italian seasoning
¼ teaspoon salt
⅛ teaspoon pepper

4 servings

In 1-quart casserole, combine peppers, onion and dressing. Cover. Microwave at High for 3 to 4 minutes, or until peppers are tender-crisp, stirring once. Set aside, covered.

In medium mixing bowl, combine remaining ingredients. Mix well. Shape into 4 patties, ½ inch thick. Place on roasting rack and cover with wax paper. Microwave at High for 4 minutes. Turn patties over and rotate rack. Re-cover. Microwave at High for another 3 to 6 minutes, or until turkey is firm.

Microwave pepper mixture at High for 1 minute, or until hot. Serve over patties.

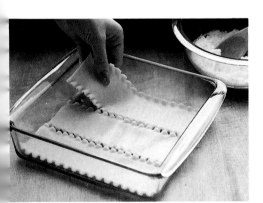

Combine ricotta, ½ cup Monterey Jack cheese and the egg in small mixing bowl. Blend well. Set aside. To assemble lasagna, cut 3 noodles to fit bottom of 9-inch square dish.

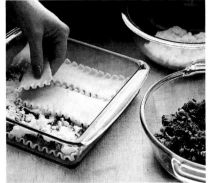

Spread one-half of meat mixture over noodles. Top with one-half of ricotta mixture and another layer of 3 noodles. Repeat once, ending with noodles. Pour reserved sauce over noodles. Sprinkle with remaining ½ cup Monterey Jack cheese.

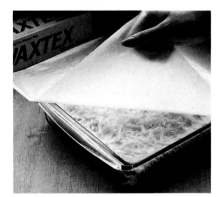

Cover with wax paper. Microwave at 70% (Medium High) for 17 to 21 minutes, or until center is hot, rotating dish once or twice. Let stand, covered, for 5 minutes. Garnish each piece with slices of cherry tomatoes, if desired.

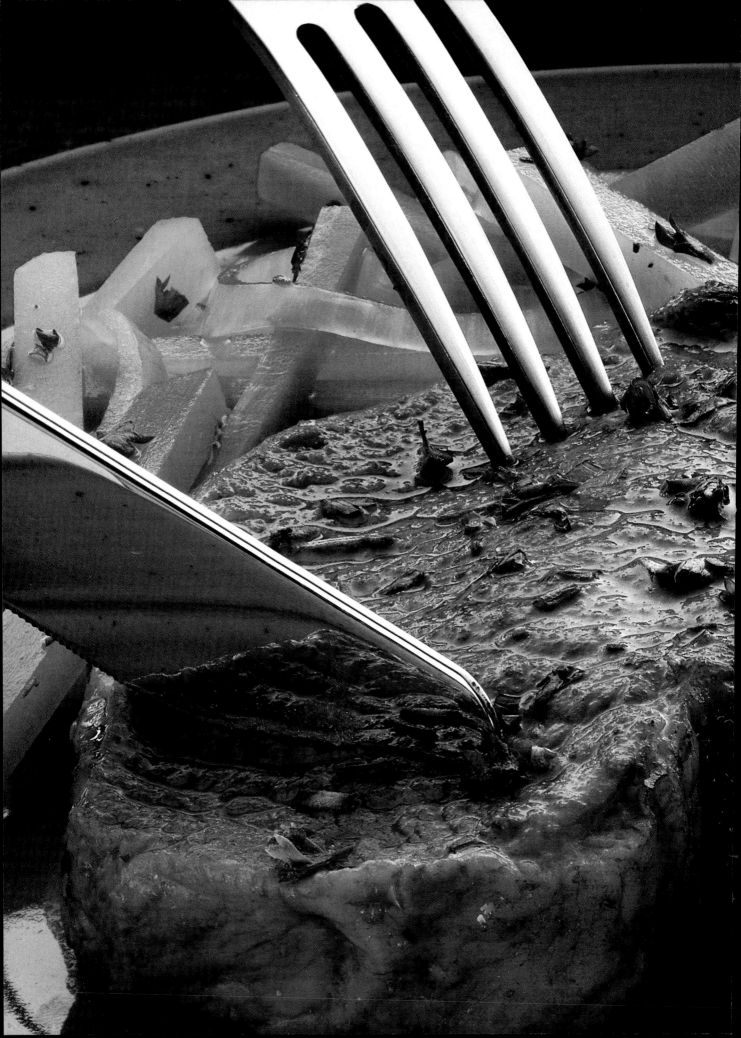

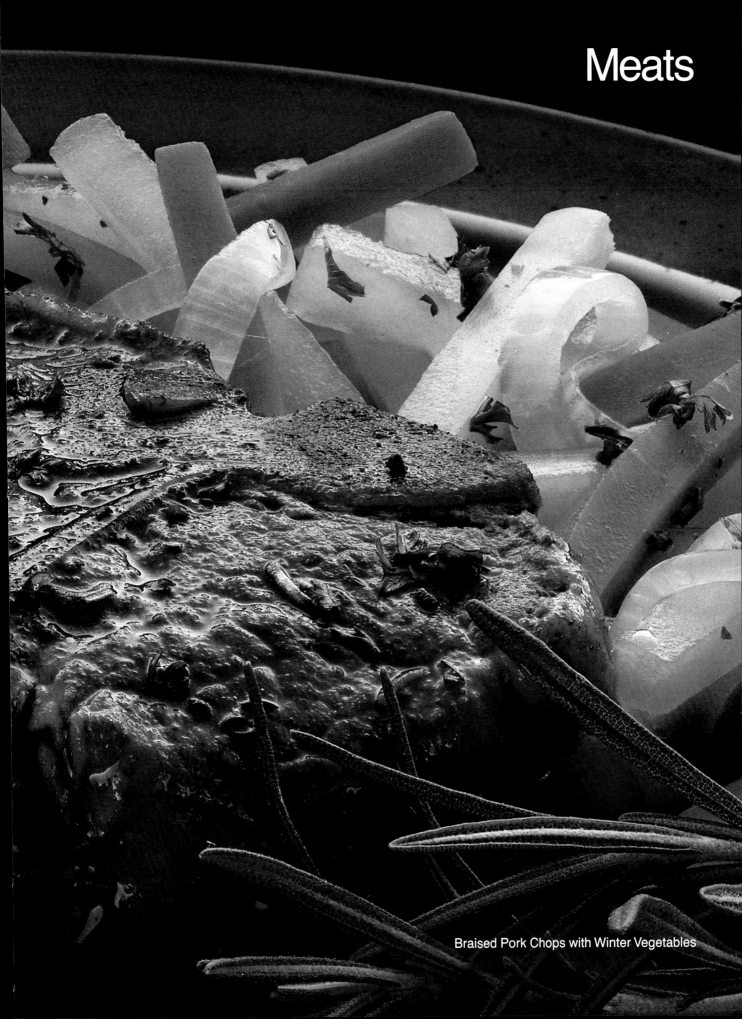

Braised Pork Chops with Winter Vegetables

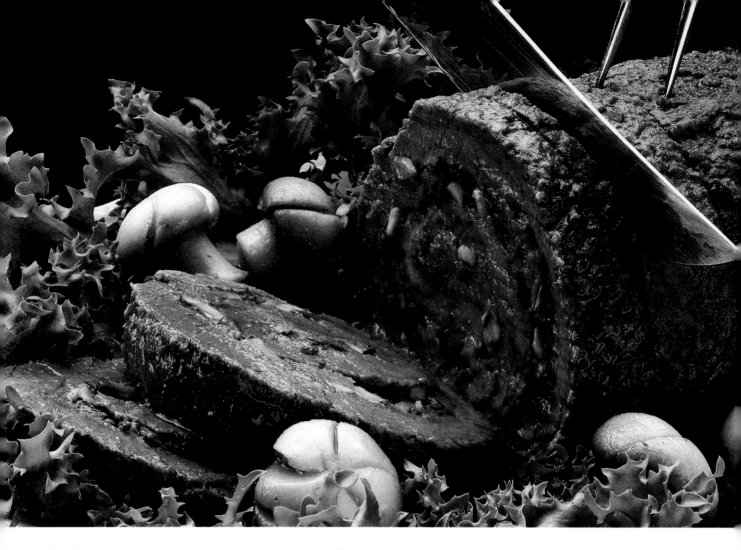

Rolled Burgundy Steak

1 to 1¼-lb. boneless beef top round steak, about ½ inch thick

Marinade:

¼ cup burgundy wine
2 tablespoons Worcestershire sauce
1 tablespoon vegetable oil
½ teaspoon dried summer savory leaves
¼ teaspoon dried tarragon leaves
¼ teaspoon coarsely ground pepper
⅛ teaspoon garlic powder

Filling:

1 cup chopped fresh mushrooms
½ cup shredded zucchini
½ cup herb-seasoned stuffing mix
⅛ teaspoon salt

4 servings

How to Microwave Rolled Burgundy Steak

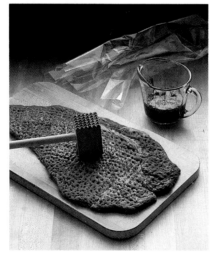

Trim steak and pound to about ¼-inch thickness. Place in nylon cooking bag. Set aside. In 1-cup measure, combine all marinade ingredients. Mix well.

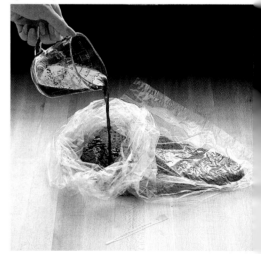

Pour marinade over steak. Secure bag with nylon tie or string. Refrigerate for at least 4 hours, or overnight. Remove meat from marinade, and lay on flat surface. Set aside. Discard marinade. Reserve bag.

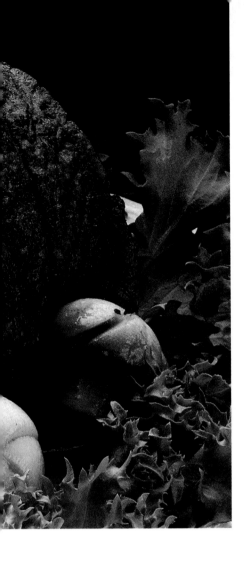

Petite Fillets with Piquant Topping

2 tablespoons sliced shallots	½ teaspoon Worcestershire sauce
1 tablespoon snipped fresh parsley	⅛ teaspoon salt Dash pepper
1 small clove garlic, minced	4 beef tenderloin steaks (4 to 5 oz. each), about 1 inch thick
1 tablespoon butter or margarine	
2 tablespoons currant jelly	
1½ teaspoons coarse brown mustard	

4 servings

In 1-quart casserole, combine shallots, parsley, garlic and butter. Microwave at High for 2 minutes. Stir in remaining ingredients except steak. Cover. Microwave at High for 1 to 2 minutes, or until jelly melts, stirring once. Set aside.

Preheat a microwave browning grill at High as directed by manufacturer. Add steaks. Let stand for 1½ minutes. Turn steaks over. Microwave at High for 3 to 4 minutes, or until beef is medium rare. Spoon topping over each steak. Serve on toasted French bread slices, if desired.

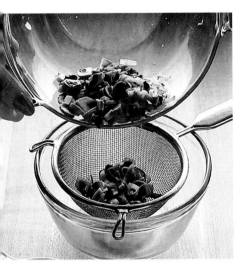

Combine mushrooms and zucchini in 1-quart casserole. Cover. Microwave at High for 3 minutes. Drain thoroughly, pressing to remove excess moisture. Return to casserole, and stir in stuffing mix and salt.

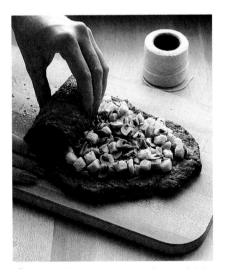

Spoon filling over steak to within ½ inch of edges, pressing lightly so filling adheres to meat. Starting with narrow end, roll up steak, enclosing filling. Tie steak in several places with string. Return steak to bag. Secure bag loosely with nylon tie or string.

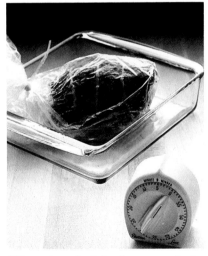

Place bag in 9-inch square baking dish. Microwave at High for 5 minutes. Microwave at 50% (Medium) for 15 to 20 minutes longer, or until beef is tender, turning over once. Let bag stand, closed, for 5 to 10 minutes. To serve steak, cut into slices.

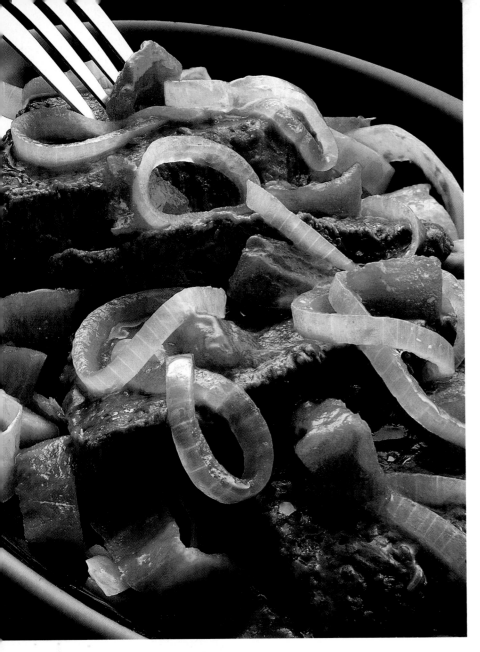

Orange Beef & Bok Choy ▶

- ¼ cup teriyaki sauce
- 2 tablespoons orange juice
- 2 tablespoons sliced green onion
- 1 clove garlic, minced
- 1 teaspoon vegetable oil
- ¼ teaspoon sesame oil (optional)
- ¼ teaspoon sugar
- ¾- lb. boneless beef sirloin steak, about 1-inch thick, cut into thin strips
- 2 cups sliced bok choy, stems and leaves, 1-inch slices
- 1 can (8 oz.) sliced water chestnuts, rinsed and drained
- 1½ teaspoons cornstarch
- ½ small orange, quartered and thinly sliced

4 servings

In 2-quart casserole, combine teriyaki sauce, orange juice, onion, garlic, oils and sugar. Microwave at High for 1 minute or until mixture is warm. Add beef strips. Let stand for 15 minutes.

Add bok choy and water chestnuts. Microwave at High for 5 to 8 minutes, or until beef is no longer pink, stirring twice. Drain liquid from beef mixture and place in 2-cup measure. Add small amount of reserved liquid to cornstarch. Blend. Add back to reserved liquid, stirring to combine. Microwave at High for 1 to 2 minutes, or until mixture is thickened and translucent, stirring every minute. Pour over beef mixture. Toss to coat. Garnish with orange slices. Serve with hot cooked rice, if desired.

Braised Beef & Cabbage Dinner ▲

- 1½- lb. boneless beef top round steak, ½ to ¾ inch thick
- 2 tablespoons all-purpose flour
- 2 teaspoons instant beef bouillon granules
- ½ teaspoon fennel seed
- ¼ teaspoon pepper
- 1 cup tomato juice
- 1 lb. cabbage, cut into ½-inch slices
- 1 small onion, thinly sliced
- 1 large tomato, peeled, seeded and chopped

4 servings

Trim steak and pound to about ¼-inch thickness. Cut into serving-size pieces. Set aside. In nylon cooking bag, place flour, beef bouillon granules, fennel and pepper. Add steak pieces. Shake to coat evenly. Pour tomato juice over steak. Add cabbage and onion.

Secure bag loosely with nylon tie or string. Place bag in 9-inch square baking dish. Microwave at High for 5 minutes. Microwave at 50% (Medium) for 35 to 45 minutes longer, or until beef is tender, turning bag over once. Add tomato. Let bag stand, closed, for 5 minutes.

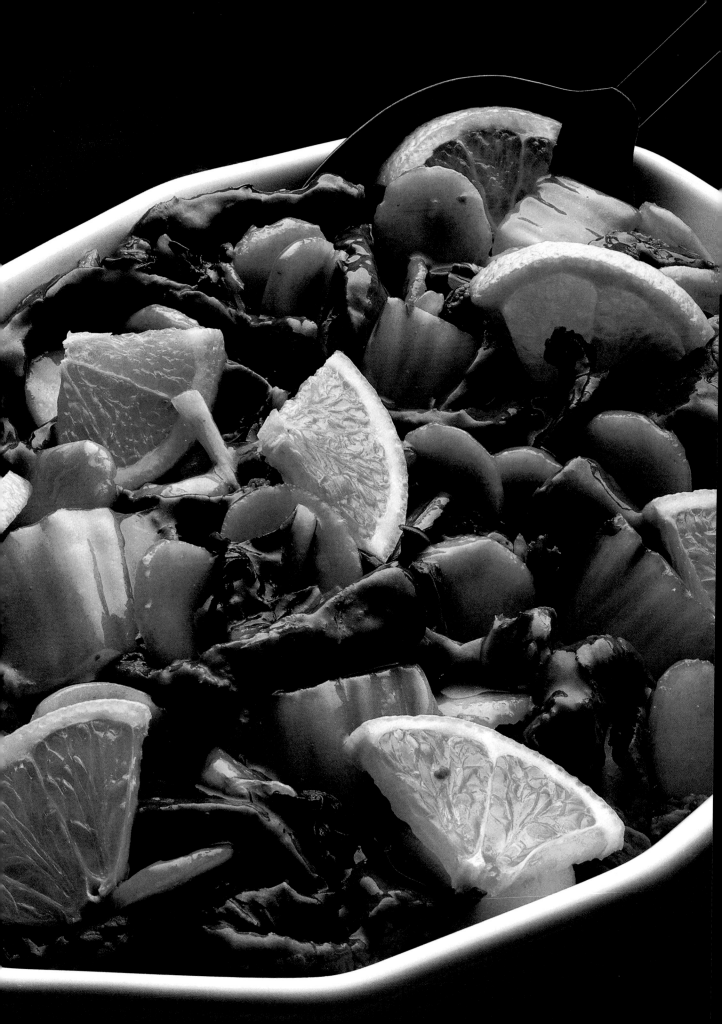

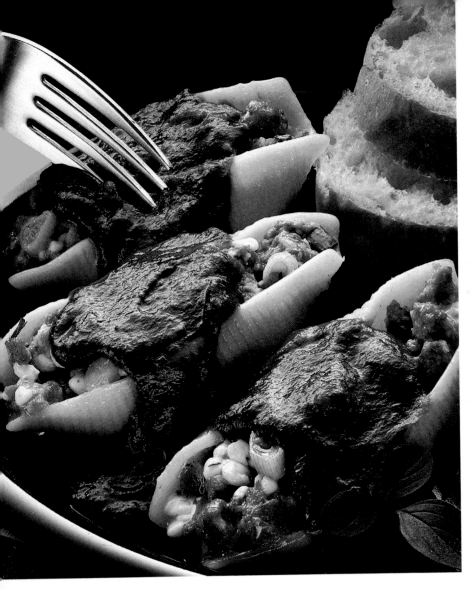

Meatloaf with Broccoli Sauce

Meatloaf:
- 1 lb. lean ground beef
- 1 cup cooked brown rice
- ¼ cup finely chopped onion
- 1 egg, beaten
- 2 tablespoons milk
- ½ teaspoon salt
- ¼ teaspoon pepper
- ⅛ teaspoon garlic powder
- ⅛ teaspoon ground nutmeg

Sauce:
- 1 cup chopped fresh broccoli
- 2 tablespoons butter or margarine
- 1 tablespoon all-purpose flour
- ¼ teaspoon salt
- ¾ cup milk
- ¼ cup shredded Swiss cheese (optional)

6 servings

In medium mixing bowl, combine all meatloaf ingredients. Mix well. Shape into 6½ × 3½-inch loaf, and place on roasting rack. Cover with wax paper. Microwave at High for 13 to 17 minutes, or until meatloaf is firm and internal temperature in center registers 150°F, rotating rack once or twice. Set aside, covered.

In 1-quart casserole, combine broccoli and butter. Cover. Microwave at High for 2½ to 3 minutes, or until broccoli is tender-crisp. Stir in flour and salt. Blend in milk. Microwave, uncovered, at High for 3 to 4½ minutes, or until sauce thickens and bubbles, stirring twice. Stir in cheese until melted. Slice meatloaf and spoon sauce over slices.

Italian Style Stuffed Shells ▲

- 12 uncooked jumbo pasta shells
- ½ lb. lean ground beef
- 1 tablespoon sliced green onion
- 1 tablespoon snipped fresh parsley, divided
- ¾ teaspoon Italian seasoning, divided
- ½ cup low-fat cottage cheese
- ¼ cup grated Parmesan cheese
- 1 egg, beaten
- ¼ teaspoon salt
- ¼ teaspoon pepper, divided
- 1 can (8 oz.) tomato sauce
- ¼ teaspoon sugar

4 servings

Prepare shells as directed on package. Rinse and drain. Set aside. Crumble ground beef into 1-quart casserole. Add onion, 2 teaspoons parsley and ½ teaspoon Italian seasoning. Cover. Microwave at High for 2 to 4 minutes, or until meat is no longer pink, stirring once to break apart. Drain. Add cheeses, egg, salt and ⅛ teaspoon pepper. Mix well. Stuff shells evenly with ground beef mixture.

Place shells in 9-inch round baking dish. Set aside. In 1-cup measure, combine tomato sauce, sugar, the remaining 1 teaspoon parsley, ¼ teaspoon Italian seasoning and ⅛ teaspoon pepper. Mix well. Pour evenly over stuffed shells. Cover with plastic wrap. Microwave at High for 6 to 8 minutes, or until filling is hot, rearranging shells once.

Beef & Bulgur Stuffed Peppers

1½ cups plus 2 tablespoons water, divided
½ cup bulgur or cracked wheat
½ lb. lean ground beef
⅓ cup shredded carrot
2 tablespoons finely chopped onion
½ teaspoon dried basil leaves
½ cup shredded Monterey Jack cheese
⅓ cup frozen corn
½ teaspoon salt
⅛ teaspoon pepper
4 large red or green peppers

4 servings

Place 1½ cups water in 4-cup measure. Microwave at High for 4 to 5 minutes, or until boiling. Stir in bulgur. Cover with plastic wrap. Let stand about 30 minutes or until bulgur softens. Drain, pressing to remove excess moisture. Set aside.

Crumble ground beef into 1-quart casserole. Add carrot, onion and basil. Cover. Microwave at High for 3 to 4 minutes, or until meat is no longer pink, stirring once to break apart. Drain. Stir in bulgur, cheese, corn, salt and pepper. Mix well. Set aside.

Cut ½-inch slice from top of peppers, reserving tops. Remove seeds and membrane. Remove thin slice from bottom of each pepper to allow peppers to stand upright. Fill peppers evenly with bulgur mixture. Place upright in 9-inch round baking dish. Add remaining 2 tablespoons water around peppers. Top peppers with reserved tops. Cover with plastic wrap. Microwave at High for 10 to 15 minutes, or until peppers are tender, rotating dish once. Let stand, covered, for 5 minutes.

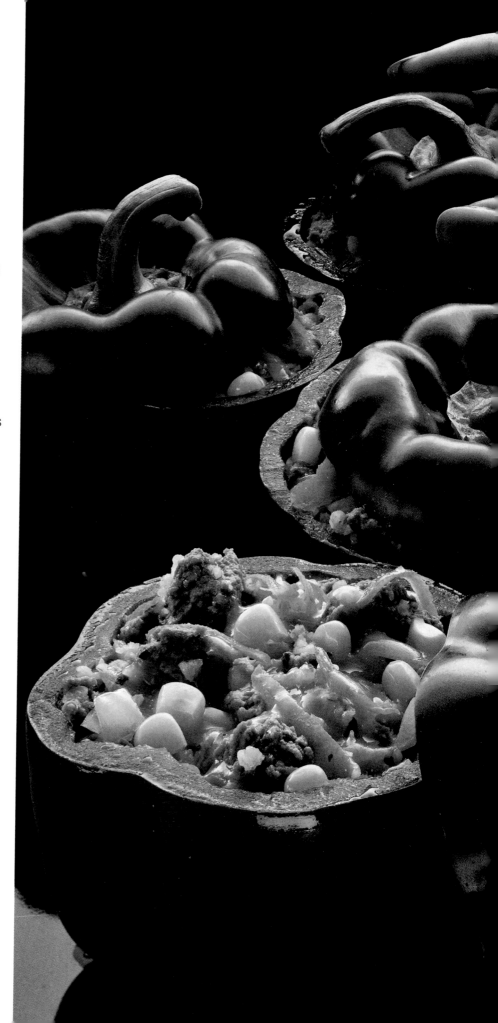

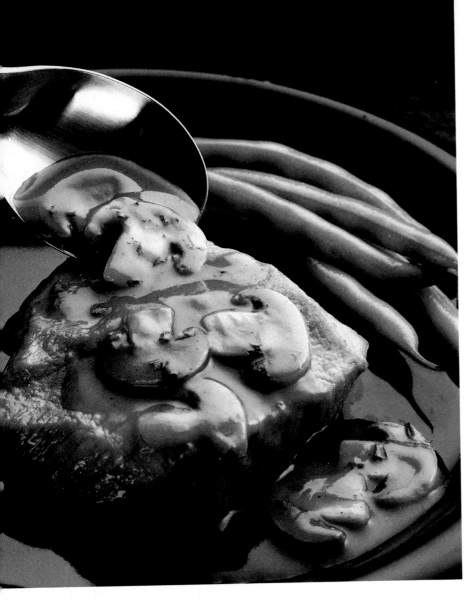

Lemon Breaded Veal with Caper Sauce

- 1 egg, beaten
- ½ cup unseasoned dry bread crumbs
- 2 teaspoons dried parsley flakes, divided
- ¾ teaspoon grated lemon peel, divided
- ½ teaspoon paprika
- ¼ teaspoon salt
- ¼ teaspoon pepper
- ¾ lb. veal scallops, about ¼ inch thick
- 2 teaspoons cornstarch
- ⅔ cup ready-to-serve chicken broth
- 2 tablespoons vermouth
- 1 teaspoon butter or margarine
- ¼ teaspoon sugar
- 1 tablespoon drained capers

4 servings

Pour egg into 9-inch pie plate. Set aside. In shallow dish, mix bread crumbs, 1 teaspoon parsley, ½ teaspoon lemon peel, the paprika, salt, and pepper. Dip veal in egg, then in crumb mixture, pressing lightly to coat both sides. Place scallops on roasting rack. Microwave at 70% (Medium High) for 7 to 10 minutes, or until veal is firm, rotating rack twice. Cover to keep warm. Set aside.

In 2-cup measure, combine remaining 1 teaspoon parsley and ¼ teaspoon lemon peel. Stir in cornstarch. Blend in broth, vermouth, butter and sugar. Microwave at High for 2½ to 4 minutes, or until mixture is thickened and translucent, stirring every minute. Add capers. To serve, pour sauce over veal.

Veal with Marsala Sauce ▲

- 1 cup sliced fresh mushrooms
- ⅓ cup ready-to-serve chicken broth
- ¼ cup sweet Marsala wine
- 2 tablespoons snipped fresh parsley
- ¼ teaspoon salt
- 1 lb. boneless veal shoulder steak, about ½ inch thick, cut into 4 serving-size pieces
- 1 tablespoon all-purpose flour
- 2 tablespoons milk
- ¼ teaspoon bouquet sauce

4 servings

In 9-inch square baking dish, combine mushrooms, broth, wine, parsley and salt. Cover with plastic wrap. Microwave at High for 4 to 5 minutes, or until mushrooms are tender, stirring once. Add veal pieces. Turn to coat with broth mixture. Re-cover. Microwave at 70% (Medium High) for 5 to 6 minutes, or until veal is medium done, rearranging pieces once. Remove veal from broth mixture. Cover veal to keep warm. Set veal and broth aside.

Place flour in small mixing bowl. Blend in milk and bouquet sauce until mixture is smooth. Add to broth mixture. Mix well. Microwave at High for 3 to 5 minutes, or until sauce thickens and bubbles, stirring every minute. To serve, pour sauce over veal.

Saucy Dijon Veal

- 1 pkg. (10 oz.) frozen asparagus cuts
- ¾ to 1-lb. boneless veal round steak, cut into ¾-inch pieces
- 3 tablespoons all-purpose flour
- ½ teaspoon salt
- ¼ teaspoon bouquet garni seasoning
- ½ cup julienne carrot (1½ × ¼-inch strips)
- ½ cup chopped onion
- 1 tablespoon butter or margarine
- 1 cup fresh mushroom halves
- ½ cup ready-to-serve chicken broth
- ⅓ cup white wine
- 2 teaspoons Dijon mustard

4 to 6 servings

Unwrap asparagus and place on plate. Microwave at High for 4 to 6 minutes, or until defrosted. Drain and set aside. Place veal pieces in large plastic food-storage bag. Add flour, salt and bouquet garni seasoning. Shake to coat meat. Set aside.

In 2-quart casserole, combine carrot, onion and butter. Cover. Microwave at High for 5 to 6 minutes, or until vegetables are tender, stirring once. Add veal and any excess flour mixture. Stir in mushrooms, broth, wine and mustard. Re-cover. Microwave at 70% (Medium High) for 13 to 16 minutes, or until veal is no longer pink, stirring twice. Add asparagus. Re-cover. Microwave at 70% (Medium High) for 4 minutes. Let stand, covered, for 10 minutes. Serve over hot cooked egg noodles, if desired.

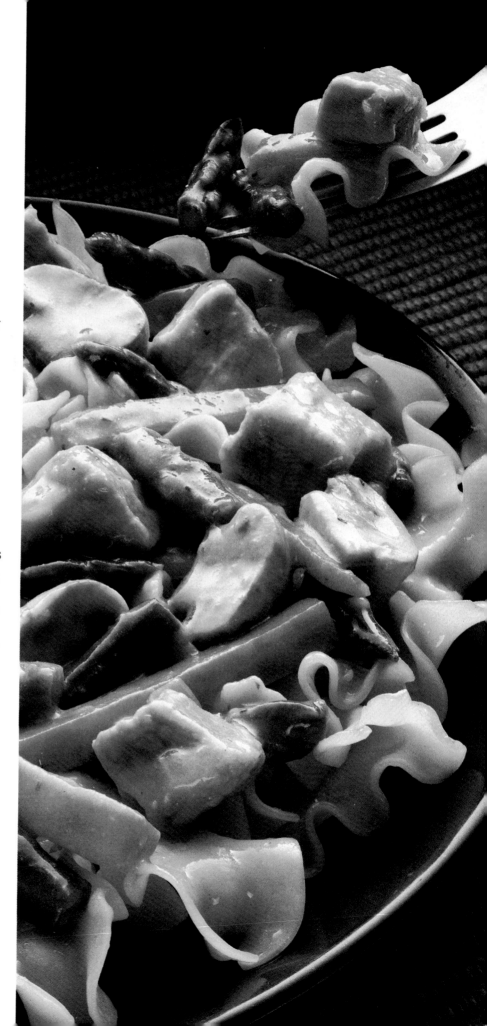

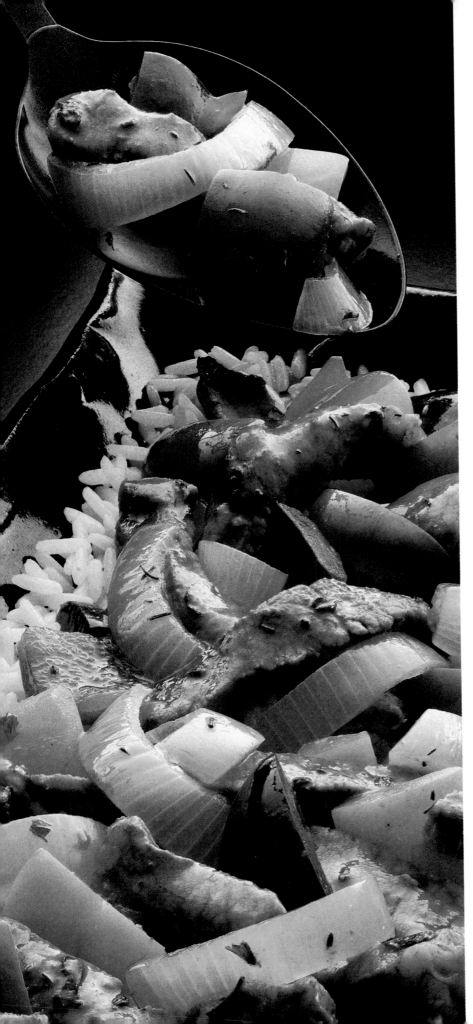

Herbed Pork & Peppers

1 medium onion, cut in half
   lengthwise and then into
   ½-inch strips
⅓ cup white wine
1 tablespoon vegetable oil
1 clove garlic, minced
½ teaspoon dried thyme leaves
½ teaspoon dried parsley flakes
¼ teaspoon salt
¼ teaspoon bouquet sauce
2 butterflied pork chops (about
   ¾ lb.), cut into ¼-inch strips
2 cups green, red or yellow
   pepper chunks (1-inch
   chunks)
1 teaspoon cornstarch

4 servings

In 2-quart casserole, combine all
ingredients, except pork, peppers
and cornstarch. Cover. Microwave
at High for 4 to 5 minutes, or until
onion is tender-crisp, stirring once.
Cool slightly. Add pork strips. Re-
cover. Refrigerate for 30 minutes
to 1 hour. Add peppers. Mix well.
Re-cover. Microwave at 70%
(Medium High) for 6 to 11 minutes, or until pork is no longer
pink, stirring once or twice.

Drain liquid from pork and peppers into a 2-cup measure. Cover
pork and peppers to keep warm.
Add a small amount of reserved
liquid to cornstarch. Blend. Add
back to reserved liquid, stirring
to combine. Microwave at High
for 1½ to 2 minutes, or until mixture is thickened and translucent,
stirring every minute. Pour over
pork and peppers. Toss to coat.
Serve with hot cooked rice or
noodles, if desired.

Braised Pork Chops with Winter Vegetables ▶

¾ cup julienne carrot
   (2 × ¼-inch strips)
¾ cup julienne rutabaga
   (2 × ¼-inch strips)
¾ cup julienne turnip
   (2 × ¼-inch strips)
1 small onion, thinly sliced
¼ cup plus 3 tablespoons
   ready-to-serve beef broth,
   divided
4 pork loin chops (5 to 6 oz.
   each), about ½ inch thick
1 tablespoon snipped fresh
   parsley
2 teaspoons packed brown
   sugar
¼ teaspoon dried rosemary
   leaves, crushed
¼ teaspoon salt
   Dash pepper

4 servings

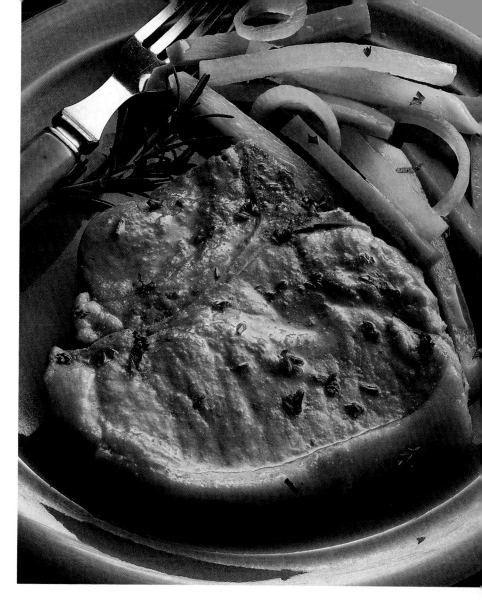

In 9-inch square baking dish, combine carrot, rutabaga, turnip and onion. Pour 3 tablespoons broth over vegetables. Cover with plastic wrap. Microwave at High for 8 to 10 minutes, or until vegetables are tender-crisp, stirring once. Arrange pork chops over vegetables, bone side toward center of dish. Set aside, covered.

In 1-cup measure, combine remaining ¼ cup broth, the parsley, brown sugar, rosemary, salt and pepper. Mix well. Pour evenly over pork chops. Re-cover. Microwave at 70% (Medium High) for 12 to 16 minutes, or until pork near bone is no longer pink, rotating dish once or twice. Let stand, covered, for 5 minutes. With slotted spoon, lift meat and vegetables to serving plate.

Plum-sauced Pork Medallions

1½ lbs. pork tenderloins,
   trimmed, diagonally sliced
   ½ inch thick
1 bay leaf
1 can (16½ oz.) whole purple
   plums, in heavy syrup
¼ cup port wine

¼ cup raisins
1½ teaspoons instant beef
   bouillon granules
½ teaspoon caraway seed
¼ teaspoon salt
⅛ teaspoon pepper

6 servings

Place tenderloin slices in 9-inch square baking dish. Add bay leaf. Set aside. Drain plums and reserve ¼ cup syrup. Remove and discard pits from plums, and place plums in food processor or blender. Process until smooth.

Place processed plums in small mixing bowl. Add reserved syrup, and remaining ingredients. Mix well. Pour over pork slices. Cover with wax paper. Microwave at 70% (Medium High) for 18 to 23 minutes, or until pork is firm and cooked through, stirring sauce and rearranging pork, 2 or 3 times. Let stand, covered, for 5 minutes. Arrange on serving plate. Spoon sauce over pork.

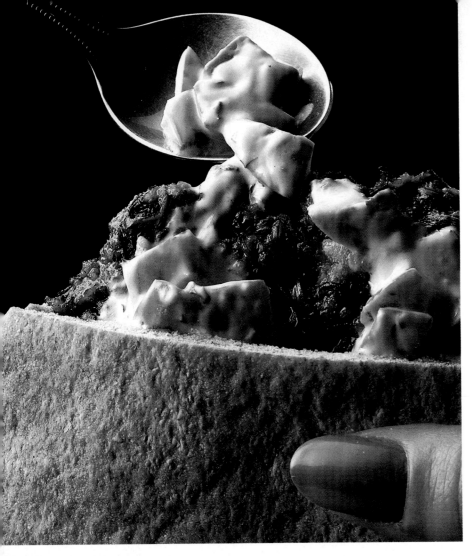

Lamb & Spinach Patties

Patties:
- 1 pkg. (10 oz.) frozen chopped spinach
- ½ lb. ground lamb
- ⅓ cup seasoned dry bread crumbs
- 1 egg, beaten
- 2 tablespoons finely chopped onion
- ½ teaspoon dried mint flakes
- ¼ teaspoon salt
- ¼ teaspoon ground cinnamon
- ¼ teaspoon ground cumin
- ⅛ teaspoon garlic powder

Topping:
- ½ cup seeded chopped tomato
- ⅓ cup plain yogurt
- ½ teaspoon dried parsley flakes
- ⅛ teaspoon garlic powder

4 servings

How to Microwave Lamb & Spinach Patties

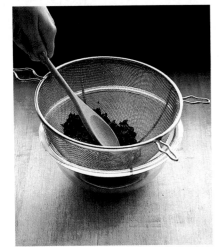

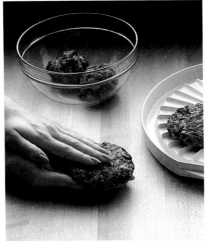

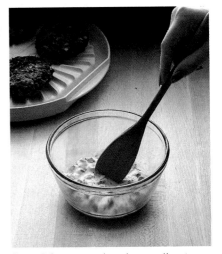

Unwrap spinach and place on plate. Microwave at High for 4 to 6 minutes, or until defrosted. Drain, pressing to remove excess moisture. Combine spinach and remaining patty ingredients in medium mixing bowl.

Shape mixture into 4 patties, ½ inch thick. Arrange on roasting rack. Cover with wax paper. Microwave at High for 5 to 6 minutes, or until meat is firm and no longer pink, rotating rack twice.

Combine topping ingredients in small mixing bowl. Mix well. Serve patties with topping. Patties may be served in pita loaves, if desired.

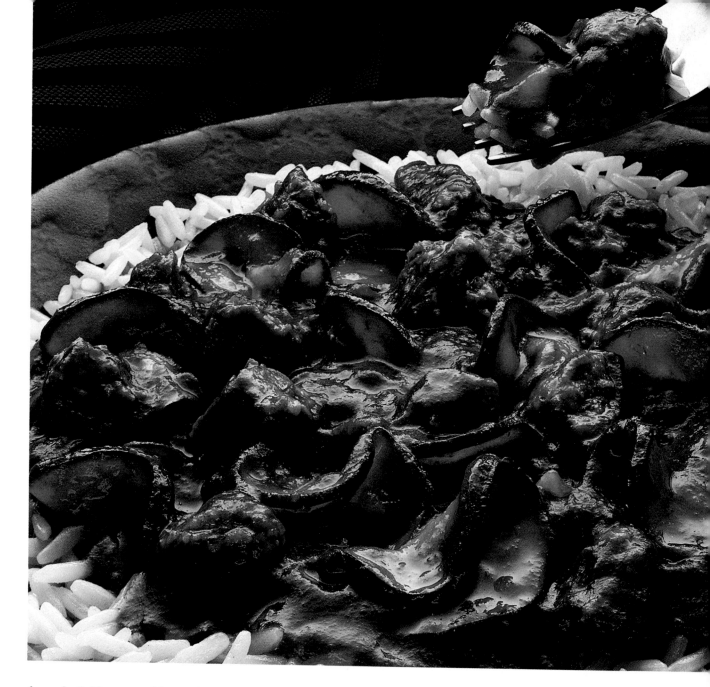

Lamb & Tomato Meat Sauce

½ lb. ground lamb
¼ cup chopped onion
1 clove garlic, minced
1 medium zucchini, thinly
    sliced
1 can (16 oz.) stewed tomatoes
1 can (8 oz.) tomato sauce
½ teaspoon dried marjoram
    leaves
¼ teaspoon dried oregano
    leaves
¼ teaspoon salt
¼ teaspoon sugar
    Hot cooked rice or noodles

4 to 6 servings

In 2-quart casserole, combine ground lamb, onion and garlic. Micro-wave at High for 2½ to 4 minutes, or until meat is no longer pink, stirring once to break apart. Drain.

Add remaining ingredients, except noodles. Cover with wax paper. Microwave at High for 10 to 14 minutes, or until sauce is hot and bubbly and zucchini is tender, stirring 2 or 3 times. Let stand, covered, for 5 minutes. Serve sauce over rice.

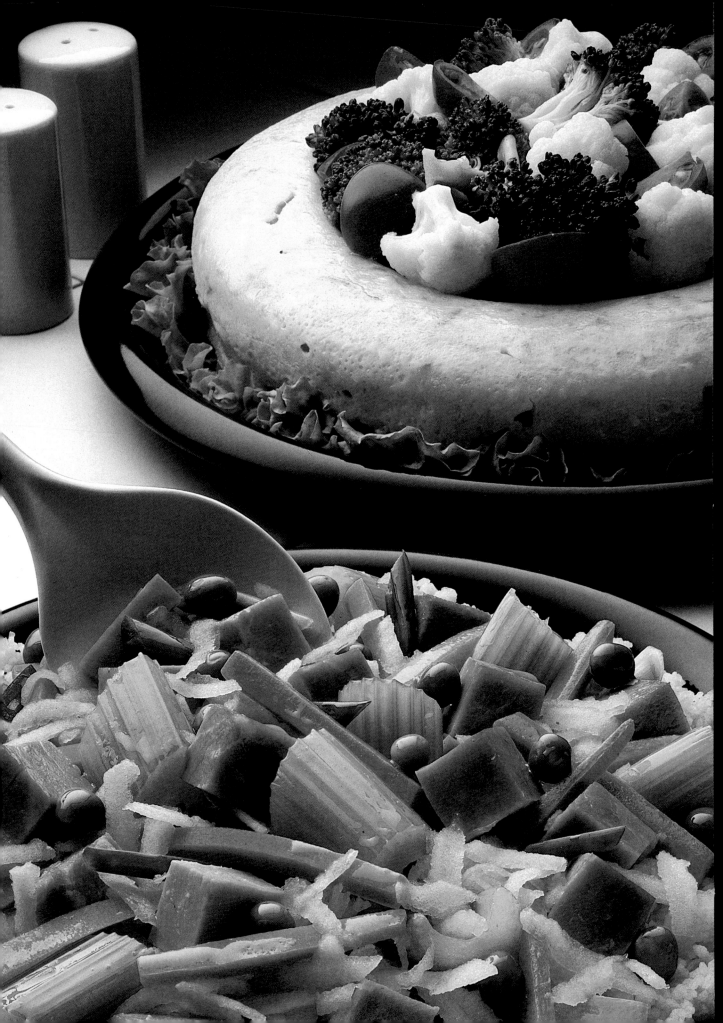

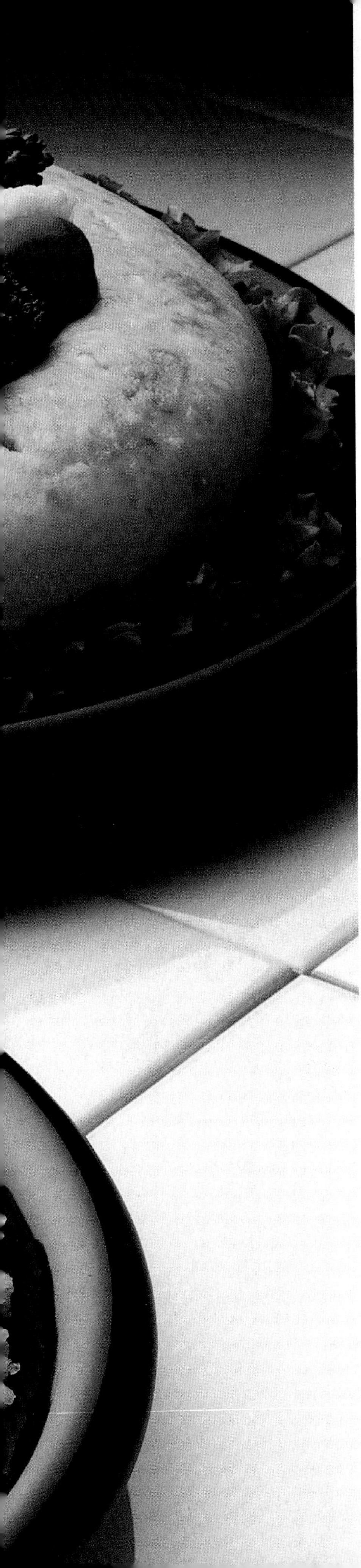

◄ Canadian Bacon Brunch Ring

Vegetable cooking spray	⅛ teaspoon pepper
4 oz. Canadian bacon slices, chopped	⅛ teaspoon dried thyme leaves
1¼ cups soft bread crumbs	1½ cups fresh broccoli flowerets
⅔ cup shredded Swiss cheese	1½ cups fresh cauliflowerets
1½ teaspoons instant minced onion	2 tablespoons water
1 can (12 oz.) evaporated skimmed milk	¼ cup quartered cherry tomatoes
5 eggs, beaten	1 tablespoon butter or margarine, cut up
¼ teaspoon salt	

6 servings

Spray 9-inch ring dish with vegetable cooking spray. Set aside. In small mixing bowl, combine Canadian bacon, bread crumbs, cheese and onion. Mix well. Spoon evenly into prepared ring dish. Set aside.

In 4-cup measure, combine milk, eggs, salt, pepper and thyme. Mix well. Pour evenly over bread crumb mixture. Cover with wax paper. Microwave at 50% (Medium) for 15 to 25 minutes, or until set and knife inserted in center comes out clean, rotating dish twice. Set aside.

In 1-quart casserole, combine broccoli, cauliflower and water. Cover. Microwave at High for 4 to 6 minutes, or until vegetables are tender-crisp, stirring once. Drain. Add tomatoes and butter. Mix well. Set aside. Loosen edges of egg mixture from sides of ring dish, and invert onto serving plate. Spoon vegetables into center.

◄ Spiced Ham with Vegetables & Couscous

1 medium cooking apple, cored, peeled and shredded	1 cup ready-to-serve chicken broth
2 medium carrots, cut into julienne strips (2 × ¼-inch)	1 stick cinnamon
	¼ teaspoon cayenne
½ cup diagonally sliced celery (1-inch slices)	¼ teaspoon curry powder
	½ lb. fully cooked ham, cut into ½-inch cubes
4 green onions, diagonally sliced (1-inch slices)	½ cup frozen peas
	1 cup uncooked couscous

4 to 6 servings

In 2-quart casserole, combine apple, carrots, celery, onions, broth, cinnamon, cayenne and curry powder. Cover. Microwave at High for 14 to 20 minutes, or until carrots and celery are tender, stirring 2 or 3 times.

Add ham and peas. Re-cover. Microwave at High for 2 minutes. Let stand, covered, for 5 minutes. Prepare couscous as directed on package. Serve ham and vegetable mixture over hot cooked couscous.

Nutrition Chart

This analysis does not include variations, optional ingredients or garnishes. Dashes indicate amounts less than 1 gram. For more complete explanation of the analysis, see page 5.

PAGE NUMBER AND RECIPE NAME	CALORIES	PROTEIN (g)	CARBOHYDRATE (g)	FAT (g)	SODIUM (mg)
8 Broccoli Cheese Dip	54	3	1	4	158
8 Bean & Salsa Dip	57	4	9	1	83
9 Cucumber Dip	31	1	2	2	101
9 Hummus	39	2	6	1	2
11 3-Cheese Spinach Dip	53	3	2	4	174
11 Spicy & Chunky Fresh Dip	8	—	2	—	129
11 Gouda Cheese Fondue	144	9	4	9	271
12 Indian Fruit Dip Platter	284	5	23	20	189
13 Hot Ham-n-Cheese Crackers	76	3	6	5	150
13 Chopped Chicken Liver Spread	75	4	2	6	127
14 Eggplant & Pepper Pita Canapés	114	3	13	6	273
14 Pizza Bread Sticks	97	6	12	3	392
15 Mediterranean Snack Platter	99	4	10	5	402
16 Marinated Vegetable Arrangement	100	1	4	10	122
17 Pesto & Cheese Tomatoes	44	3	2	3	48
17 Cocktail Snacks	32	1	2	2	199
18 Cheesy Bacon Skins	270	8	14	21	221
19 Pizza Potato Skins	230	7	16	16	350
19 Cream Cheese & Shrimp-topped Skins	300	13	15	21	188
19 Herb Chicken Potato Skins	314	14	15	22	379
20 Snack Pizza Crust	232	7	33	8	468
20 Pizza Sauce	32	1	7	—	106
21 Artichoke & Pepper Pizza	471	16	49	25	894
21 Tuna & Olive Pizza	423	26	42	17	726
22 Turkey & Fresh Basil Pizza	418	24	43	17	711
22 Prosciutto & Mushroom Pizza	406	21	42	18	1164
23 Summertime Pizza	346	16	43	13	727
23 Shrimp & Bacon Pizza	487	26	41	25	1030
24 South of the Border Cheese Crisp	132	7	6	9	242
25 Fresh Vegetable Cheese Crisp	106	3	6	8	90
27 Spicy Sesame Marinade and Wings	87	9	3	4	519
27 Orange Barbecue Marinade and Wings	77	8	7	2	253
27 Hot Garlic Marinade and Wings	70	9	5	2	339
27 Dipping Sauce	62	—	1	7	73
28 Chicken & Broccoli Bites	123	15	8	4	820
30 Pea-Pod-wrapped Shrimp	64	8	2	3	567
31 Shrimp & Pepper Kabobs	82	7	2	5	129
31 Shrimp Cocktail	108	12	11	2	547
32 Cheesy Mexican Popcorn	128	2	5	11	243
32 Sour Cream Chive Popcorn	87	1	6	7	91
32 Herb Parmesan Popcorn	128	3	5	11	263
33 Crunchy Snack Mix	502	11	37	36	712
33 Seasoned Sticks & Stones	339	7	21	27	240
33 Hot Soft Pretzels	133	5	17	5	340
35 Mexican Hot Chocolate	191	7	34	5	134
35 Hot Pineapple Punch	111	1	19	4	40
35 Hot Bloody Mary	75	2	10	—	1016
35 Hearty Health Broth	31	4	5	—	706
36 Cardamom-Spice Coffee	57	2	8	2	34

PAGE NUMBER AND RECIPE NAME	CALORIES	PROTEIN (g)	CARBOHYDRATE (g)	FAT (g)	SODIUM (mg)
36 Gingered Orange Tea	13	—	3	—	2
36 Peachy Iced Tea	33	—	9	—	2
36 Lemon & Spice Tea	1	—	—	—	1
37 Strawberry Margaritas	268	—	50	—	2
37 Refreshing Lime Cooler	123	—	32	—	1
37 Tangy Raspberry Shake	183	6	36	2	127
40 Mandarin Orange Sauce	40	—	8	1	13
40 Ginger-spiced Applesauce	69	—	18	—	1
40 Rhubarb & Raspberry Dessert Sauce	34	—	9	—	3
41 Pudding & Yogurt Cones	200	6	36	4	164
41 Banana Macaroon Gratin	326	5	53	13	115
42 Ruby Red Pears	216	—	39	—	3
43 Custard Sauce & Mixed Fruit	273	8	52	4	124
45 Crispy Fruit & Cheese Rounds	186	4	21	10	122
45 Mini Savarins	231	3	48	3	68
45 Mexican Apple Strudel	313	2	64	7	134
45 Fresh Fruit Compote	123	1	30	1	7
46 Lemon Blueberry Mousse	98	4	15	3	48
47 Raspberry Bavarian	88	1	10	5	79
48 Fluffy Strawberry Layers	116	2	19	4	7
49 Orange-Pineapple Snowballs	68	—	17	—	1
49 Gingersnap-Apricot Freeze	162	4	23	6	168
50 Strawberry-Cheese Dessert	267	4	24	18	205
50 Yogurt & Fruit Candy Bars	74	1	16	1	48
51 Crunchy Granola	141	2	24	5	19
54 Apple-Ginger Fruit Salad	110	1	27	1	18
55 Confetti Rice Salad	266	5	35	13	219
55 Fresh Green Bean Salad	230	6	11	19	349
56 Festive Turkey Rice Salad	237	8	26	12	205
56 Chicken Taco Salad	284	33	11	11	203
57 Chicken Platter with Orange-Basil Dressing	375	31	6	25	333
59 Oriental Shrimp & Pasta Salad	381	17	56	10	592
59 Creamy Tortellini & Salmon Salad	382	14	23	27	356
60 Bavarian Ham & Potato Salad	661	23	37	48	906
61 7-Layer Beef Salad	177	12	6	12	238
61 Tossed Garden Salad with Sirloin	148	10	3	11	100
62 Cold Cherry Soup	103	2	21	1	45
63 Creamy Italian Summer Squash Soup	106	4	10	6	307
63 Ginger Carrot Soup	187	5	20	10	758
64 Creamy Leek Soup	194	5	18	12	843
64 Beet Soup	76	2	10	3	566
65 Avocado Soup	185	5	7	16	630
65 Mexican Corn Chowder	155	6	19	7	870
67 Fresh Tomato Basil Soup	69	2	12	3	627
67 Vegetable-Beef Soup	272	19	36	6	373
67 Vegetable Clam Chowder	237	11	29	9	811
68 Breast of Chicken with Rice Soup	204	26	15	3	493
68 Black Bean Soup	172	11	21	5	447
69 St. Pat's Day Soup	177	7	15	11	474

PAGE NUMBER AND RECIPE NAME	CALORIES	PROTEIN (g)	CARBOHYDRATE (g)	FAT (g)	SODIUM (mg)
71 Hot Barbecue Sandwiches	291	22	28	10	678
71 Italian Sloppy Subs	502	21	47	26	1147
71 Chicken Cashew Sandwiches	354	22	26	18	495
72 Mexican Patty Melts	438	28	23	25	532
72 Mock Gyros	442	28	46	16	400
73 Philly Beef Sandwiches	499	30	41	23	948
74 Salmon Smokies	258	15	17	15	147
74 Turkey Club Pitas	275	17	23	13	563
75 Summer Vegie Melt	488	17	31	34	882
75 Triple-Cheese Sandwiches	385	16	28	24	604
78 Stuffed Cheese Potatoes	473	17	44	27	677
79 Zesty Stuffed Potatoes	348	12	43	15	373
80 Vegetable-topped Potatoes	396	16	64	10	700
81 4-Cheese Pie with Whole Wheat Crust	448	23	23	30	705
82 Cheesy Chili Enchiladas	285	11	19	18	835
83 3-Bean Chili	170	9	30	3	751
85 Mediterranean Vegetable Sauté	274	5	35	13	297
85 Curried Potato & Garden Vegetable Sauce	239	5	42	6	553
85 Fresh Vegetable Alfredo	582	19	49	36	732
86 Crunchy Wild Rice Casserole	470	21	48	22	619
86 Scalloped Vegetable Bake	425	21	29	24	781
87 Vegetable Chowder	198	9	13	13	350
88 Italian Eggplant Bake	375	17	18	27	825
90 Florentine Mostaccioli Bake	614	19	62	31	792
90 Linguine & Red-Peppered Broccoli	406	12	42	23	382
91 Vegetable Lasagna Spirals	439	24	39	21	493
94 Neptune Torte	474	31	34	23	909
96 Lemon-Dijon Fillets	131	17	4	5	223
96 Citrus-sauced Shrimp & Fillets	149	22	5	5	304
97 Fillets Florentine with Sesame Butter	211	21	1	13	220
97 Mushroom-topped Fillets	140	17	4	6	256
97 Mexican Salsa Fillets	105	16	4	3	253
99 Orange-sauced Roughy	104	13	6	—	103
99 Cod & Tomato Bake	163	15	13	6	441
99 Cajun Stuffed Sole	298	25	32	8	858
100 Poached Salmon with Sour Cream Dill Sauce	445	41	6	28	124
101 Halibut Veronique	242	32	7	8	371
101 Scandinavian Fish Patties	313	17	22	17	320
102 Herb-seasoned Swordfish Steaks	232	28	—	13	144
102 Easy Crab & Mushroom Dinner	187	9	24	6	655
102 Salmon-stuffed Green Pepper Rings	343	18	29	18	656
103 Tuna-stuffed Shells	364	21	35	15	849
104 Salmon Brunch Pie	372	16	17	27	560
105 Seafood Platter with Lime Poppy Seed Dressing	199	19	15	7	305
106 Garden Scallop Stuffed Tomatoes	156	16	14	4	318
107 Shrimp & Fresh Vegetable Aspic	82	10	9	1	442
108 Curried Orange Roughy & Vegetables	263	20	32	4	458
108 Linguine & Clam Bake	233	11	32	6	126
108 Saucy Creole Casserole	191	11	26	5	476
109 Saffron Shrimp & Tomatoes	164	9	28	1	251
110 Oriental Orange Seafood Kabobs	237	20	29	4	941
112 Spicy Shrimp & Pan-fried Noodles	398	21	51	12	1141
113 Scallop & Ham Bake	238	20	26	6	515
116 Savory Fruit-stuffed Cornish Game Hens	421	44	23	17	664
117 Carrot-stuffed Chicken	395	42	8	20	430
118 Lime & Cumin Cornish Game Hens	334	41	16	11	403
119 Raspberry Chicken	244	36	14	4	184
119 Orange-Mint Braised Chicken Thighs	432	30	34	18	374
120 Honey Lemon Chicken Breasts	238	36	14	4	343
121 Golden Cheddary Chicken	348	43	4	16	369
122 Chili & Chicken Burritos	409	34	42	12	630
122 Chicken & Zucchini Enchiladas	294	18	23	12	414
123 Whole Wheat Chicken & Broccoli Strata	243	20	16	12	468
124 Spicy Rice & Skewered Chicken	260	25	30	4	430
125 Warm Spanish Chicken Salad	245	18	22	9	524
127 Chicken Almond Ding	378	31	33	13	508
127 Caribbean Chicken Medley	178	25	11	4	413
127 Lemon Chicken & Broccoli with Poppy Seed Noodles	458	33	45	16	277
128 Roast Turkey with Garden Squash Stuffing	351	55	19	5	489
130 Cranberry-stuffed Turkey Tenderloins	181	28	9	3	162
131 Fresh Fruit-stuffed Turkey	256	43	16	1	163
132 Olive-topped Turkey Cutlets	129	19	1	4	280
132 Turkey Cutlets with Green Chili Sauce	235	33	11	6	653
133 Turkey Fajitas	232	24	23	5	129
133 Turkey Chili	201	20	26	2	644
134 Mediterranean Lasagna	377	27	32	15	596
135 Italian Turkey Patties	209	30	6	6	311
138 Rolled Burgundy Steak	241	29	14	7	386
139 Petite Fillets with Piquant Topping	182	18	7	9	172
140 Braised Beef & Cabbage Dinner	254	34	14	7	490
140 Orange Beef & Bok Choy	148	14	11	5	623
142 Italian Style Stuffed Shells	298	24	29	9	747
142 Meatloaf with Broccoli Sauce	239	19	12	12	372
143 Beef & Bulgur Stuffed Peppers	275	19	28	10	381
144 Veal with Marsala Sauce	230	25	3	11	245
144 Lemon Breaded Veal with Caper Sauce	241	21	11	10	436
145 Saucy Dijon Veal	188	18	8	8	370
146 Herbed Pork & Peppers	213	17	7	11	176
147 Braised Pork Chops with Winter Vegetables	310	33	9	15	318
147 Plum-sauced Pork Medallions	246	26	23	4	245
148 Lamb & Spinach Patties	147	14	10	6	319
149 Lamb & Tomato Meat Sauce	203	11	31	5	614
151 Canadian Bacon Brunch Ring	245	19	15	12	584
151 Spiced Ham with Vegetables & Couscous	173	12	25	3	612

Index